ECG/EKG INTERPRETATION

AN EASY APPROACH TO READ A 12-LEAD ECG AND HOW TO DIAGNOSE AND TREAT ARRHYTHMIAS

By

NATHAN ORWELL

Discover the Entire Collection!

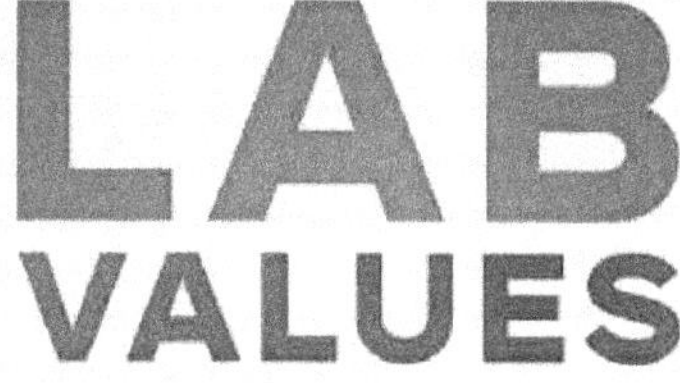

TABLE OF CONTENTS

INTRODUCTION

The electrocardiogram (EKG/ECG) is one of the foremost useful diagnostic tests in medicine. It's an easy and cheap test often utilized in the evaluation of patients with pain. The ECG is the cornerstone of the diagnosis of cardiac ischemia and is employed to form decisions about suitability for therapy. It's an image of the heart's electrical conductivity. By examining changes from normal on the ECG, doctors can identify many heart condition processes.

I hope you will enjoy this book, and that it helped you in your understanding and interpretation of ECGs.

If you'd like, you can leave a review here!

CHAPTER 1: ELECTROCARDIOGRAM (ECG)

An electrocardiogram, abbreviated as ECG or EKG, may be a test that measures the electrical activity of the heart rhythm. An electrocardiogram is a medical test that ascertains how well your heart functions by measuring the heart's electrical activity. With every heartbeat, an electrical impulse (or wave) passes through your heart. This wave causes the muscles to contract and pump blood from the heart.

The electrocardiograph (ECG or EKG for short) is a device that detects electrical activity in the body coming from the heart. Within the clinic, the ECG is one of the foremost commonly used diagnostic devices. The recording produced by the electrocardiograph is named an electrocardiogram.

ELECTROCARDIOGRAM WAVEFORM

An electrical impulse, also called a wave, passes through the heart. This wave causes the muscle to contract and pump blood from the heart. A standard heart rate on the ECG shows the timing of the upper and lower chambers of the heart.

The right and left upper chambers (atria) produce the first wave, called the "P wave," which goes through a flat line when the electrical impulse travels to the lower chambers. The right and left lower chambers or ventricles produce the next wave, the "QRS complex."

The final wave or "T wave" represents the electrical recovery or return to a resting state of the ventricles. An ECG may be suggested if you are experiencing arrhythmia or any form of heart or chest problems.

The following image shows a normal ECG. Three distinctive characteristic features of the waveform are easily recognized: the P wave, the QRS complex, and the T wave. The P wave is linked with the activation and functioning of the atria, the QRS complex is linked with the activation of the ventricles, and the T wave is linked with the repolarization of the ventricles.

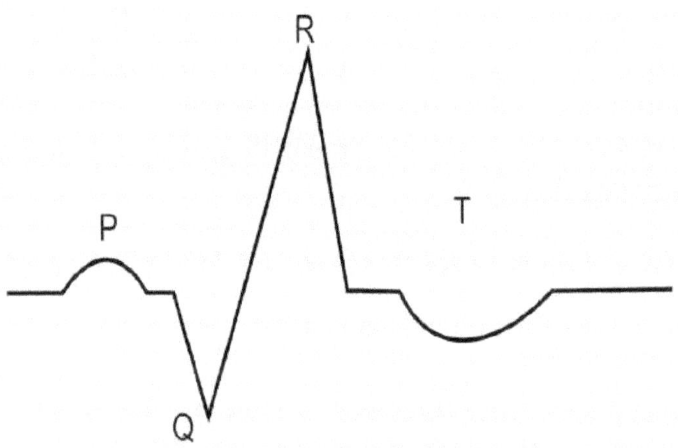

Normal ECG

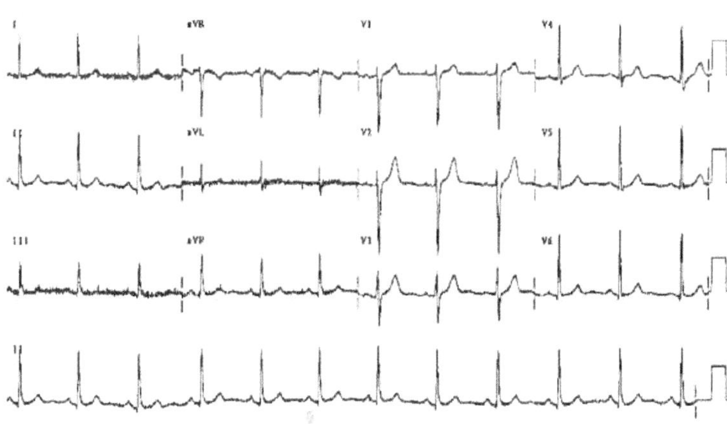

ELECTROCARDIOGRAM INTERVALS

- The interval between p-r is the time from the start of the P wave to the beginning of the Q-R-S complex.
- The Q-R-S interval (width) is the time from the beginning to the end of the Q-R-S complex.
- The Q-T interval (width) is the time frame between the Q-R-S complex and the T wave.
- The R- R interval is the time frame from the peak of one R wave and the next R wave.

ELECTROCARDIOGRAPH: TECHNICAL PRINCIPLES

The electrocardiograph is an ineluctable electronic device that amplifies the microscopic potentials on the surface of the body so that it can be displayed on a video screen or recorded on a sheet of paper. The readings are picked up by electrodes put in well-defined anatomical positions on the surface of the body.

The main part of the ECG is an electronically amplified two vital input terminals, a non-inverting (+) input terminal and an inverting (-) input terminal. The output voltage Vo is merely proportional to the difference between the V+ and V- voltages appearing on the two input terminals:

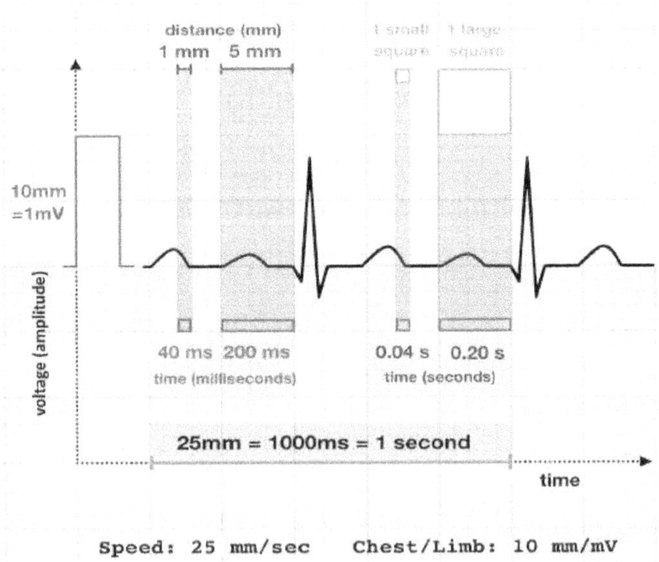

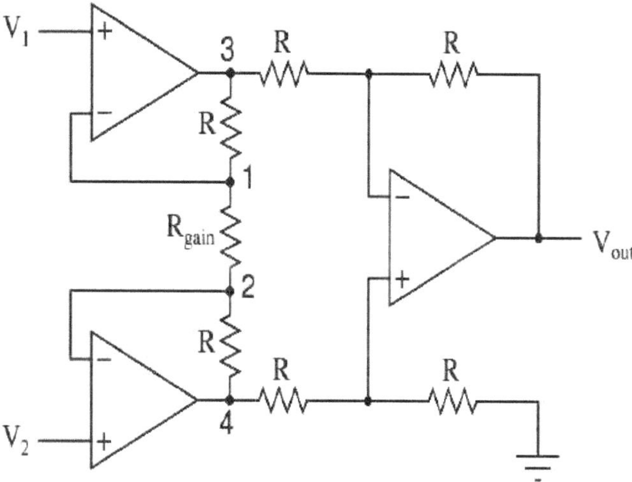

Note: R= the gain of the amplifier.

Hence, the amplifier is called a differential amplifier as it evaluates the difference between two voltages.

You will remember from your introductory physics courses that voltage or electrical potential a relative quantity in the sense that the potential itself cannot be measured. Only differ in potential. Therefore, V+ and V- are each measured with respect to a third reference point, which is arbitrarily taken as zero potential. In electrocardiography, this point is referred to as the right leg. The differential amplifier has the benefit that any part of the signal that appears simultaneously at both inputs is cancelled and thus does not appear at the output.

This "common mode rejection" is essential because 115-volt electrical wiring in a building can generate signals at 60 Hz (the frequency of the power line) on the body surface that are many times greater than the signal itself.

ECG. The use of a differential amplifier prevents this large spurious signal from flooding the ECG signal.

INTERVALS AND SEGMENTS

The PR interval shows the beginning of the P wave to the beginning of the QRS complex.

The PR segment indicates the end of the P wave to the start of the same QRS complex.

Point J is the intersection between the QRS complex and the ST segment.

The QT interval is the beginning of the QRS complex to the end of the T wave.

The QRS interval starts at the end of the QRS complex.

ST-segment: from the end of the QRS complex (point J) to the beginning of the T wave

Normal values

Heart rate 60-100 beats per minute

0.12 - 0.20 s (PR interval)

QRS interval ≤ 0.12 s

QT interval <half-life RR (men <0.40 s; women <0.44 s)

P wave amplitude (in cable II) ≤ 3 mV (mm)

STEP BY STEP APPROACH TO THE ECG

If the full ECG is 10 seconds, there should be 50 large boxes (0.20 seconds for 50 large boxes). Each small box is also exactly 1mm long; therefore, a large box is 5 mm.

In general, when measuring wave amplitudes or complexes, the units are expressed in mm, and when measuring interval lengths, the units are expressed in seconds or milliseconds (ms). If each small frame is equal to 0.04 seconds or 1 mm, the default ECG speed is 1 mm per 0.04 seconds or 25 mm per second.

The standard method of reading an ECG includes, in this order:

Step A: Ascertain the heart rate

There are numerous strategic ways of determining heart rate. A quick and easy technique is to find a QRS complex that lies on a vertical major grid line;

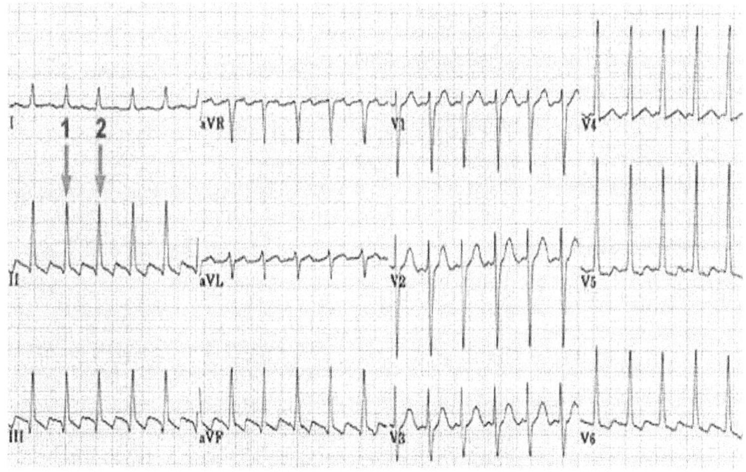

(1) Note the number of big squares to the next QRS complex

(2). Divide the number by 300, and you get the heart rate.

Step B: Measure the necessary intervals

Measurement of necessary ECG intervals usually includes the following: PR, QR, and QT intervals, respectively. At a paper speed of 26 mm/ second, the width of each square (1.5 mm) is 0.06 seconds. A large square (5 mm) represents 0.10 seconds.

Step C (i): Calculate the Electric Axis

In numerous cases, an approximation of the axis will be enough for the interpretation of the ECG. There are many different steps in ascertaining the axis, but this discussion will be limited to a simple technique that uses leads I and aVF to calculate an approximate axis. Note that the axis can be viewed regarding four quadrants, with lead I oriented at 0 ° and aVF oriented at + 90 °. An ECG with the QRS axis pointing to the quadrant between 0 ° and 90 ° would be expected.

- An ECG with the QRS axis pointing to the quadrant between -1 ° and -90 ° would have a deviation from the left axis.
- An ECG with the QRS pointing to the quadrant between + 91 ° and 180 ° would have a deviation from the right axis.

- An ECG with the QRS targeting the quadrant between -91 ° and -180 ° would have an indefinite axis because it cannot be said whether it represents a deviation from the right or left axis.

Step C (ii): Calculate the Electric Axis

The middle QRS axis faces the head with the most significant apparent QRS deviation. To calculate the net deflection of the QRS, add the number of little squares that correlate to the height of the positive deflection (R wave) and subtract the number of little squares that correspond to the height of the negative deflection (Q and S waves).

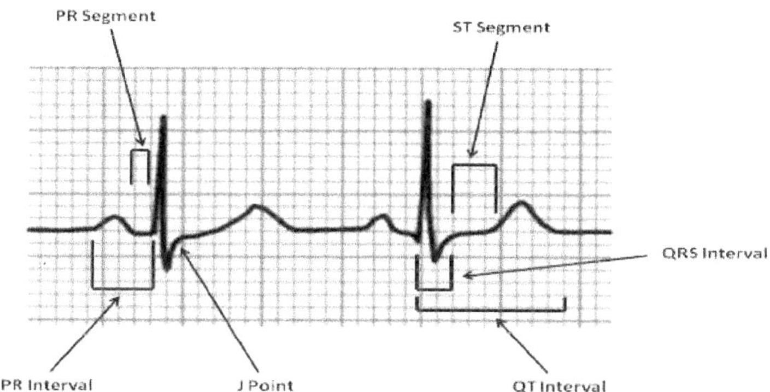

Step D: Assess the heart rate

The RR interval should be constant during the ECG reading, and it showed a regular heart rhythm. This can be verified with a calliper, or more simply by marking the distance between two R waves and comparing this distance between pairs of QRS complexes on the ECG. Then check if there is a P wave for each of the QRS complexes.

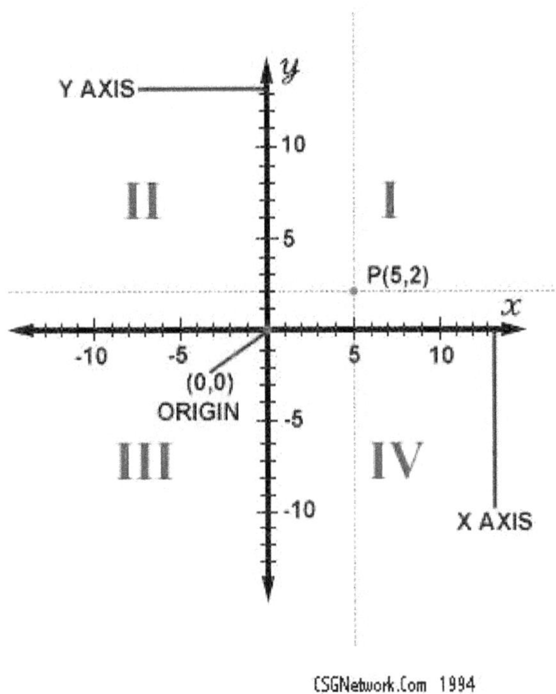

Step E: Inspect the p waves for atrial magnification.

In leads, I, II, III, and V1 (P wave) should be inspected for signs of left or right atrial magnification. Lead II generally has the lightest P wave. The amplitude of the P wave must not exceed three small squares (3 mm or 0.3 mV). If so, it represents an enlarged right atrium in Lead V1; the negative pole deviation of the P-wave represents depolarization of the left atrium and should not exceed 1 mm (0.1 mV). If so, this indicates an enlarged left atrium.

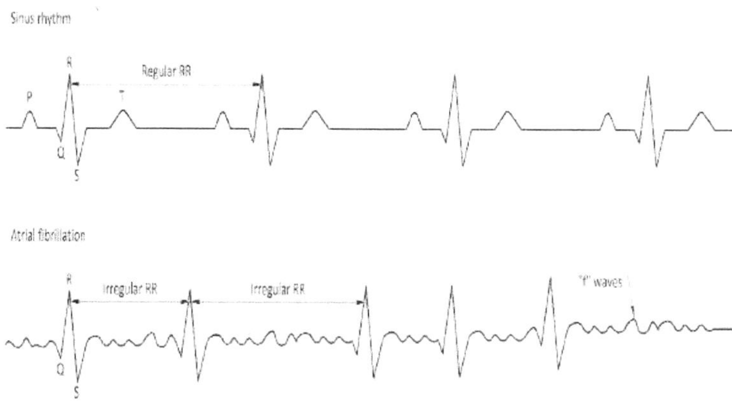

Step F: Inspect the QRS complexes for ventricular hypertrophy or low voltage

In left ventricular hypertrophy (LVH), the left ventricle dilates, and therefore the leads pointing to the left ventricle (V5, V6, aVL) will 'see' more electrical activity moving towards them. Also, leads directed away from the left ventricle (V1, V2) will see more action away from them. Therefore, in LVH, leads V5, V6 and aVL have large R waves, while leads V1 and V2 have deep S waves.

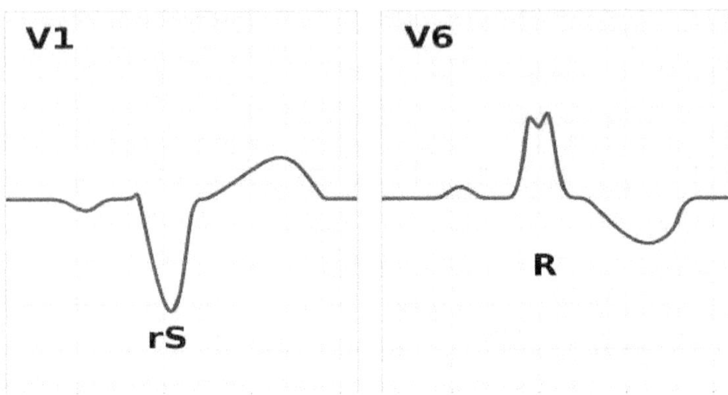

Action away from them. Therefore, in LVH, leads V5, V6 and aVL have large R waves, while leads V1 and V2 have deep S waves.

Step G (i): Inspect the QRS complexes for bundle branch block or a fascicular block

The average QRS interval is 0.12 seconds (3 mm or three small squares) on the ECG. Use the probe with the largest QRS complex to correctly determine the QRS interval. If the QRS complex < = 0.12 seconds, no further analysis is required. If it takes longer than 0.12 seconds, you should try to establish the reason for the unusually long QRS interval. A simple approach is to consider the three possible causes of QRS magnification:

Step G (ii): Inspect the QRS complexes for bundle branch block or a fascicular block

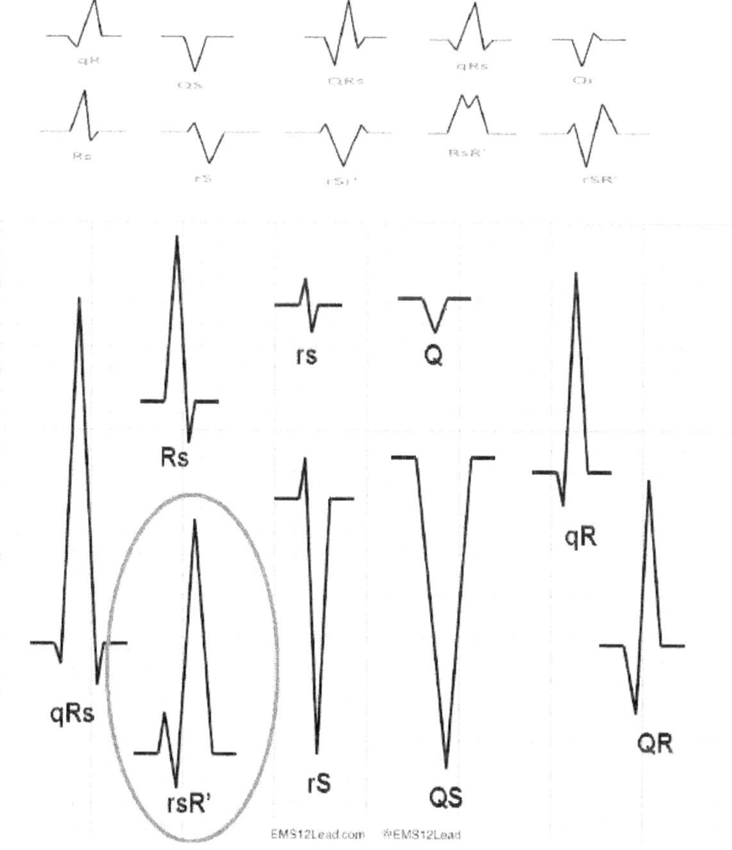

In the normal heart, at the onset of ventricular depolarization, the QRS axis is oriented to the right due to the left-to-right depolarization of the septum. This generates a small R wave in lead V1. Immediately after depolarization of the septum, then the ventricles depolarise. The size of the left ventricle results in a predominantly left axis for the rest of the QRS complex.

Step G (iii): Inspect the QRS complexes for bundle branch block or a fascicular block

In RBBB, the first part of the ECG does not change because septal depolarization and left ventricular depolarization are not affected. However, the right ventricle depolarises slowly and slowly. This emanates from an expansion of the terminal part of the QRS complex and the orientation of the axis of the QRS complex to the right.

In LBBB, there is depolarization of the right and left ventricles through the right bundle. As a result of the septum activation from right to left, the QRS axis is predominantly leftward and mainly secondary to the slow activation of the left ventricle.

Step G (iv): Inspect the QRS complexes for bundle branch block or a fascicular block

If the ECG cannot show as a typical LBBB or a typical RBBB, it can be classified as an intraventricular conduction delay. This is not discussed in more detail at this time.

Step H: Evaluate Q waves and determine their importance

Q waves must be evaluated, and their importance determined, especially concerning the diagnosis of myocardial infarction. Small Q waves are generally a normal finding in inferior leads III and aVF and in anterolateral leads aVL, I, V5, and V6. Q waves with a time range of 0.06 seconds (1 mm) and more than one-third of the volume of the R wave in the same probe can be pathological.

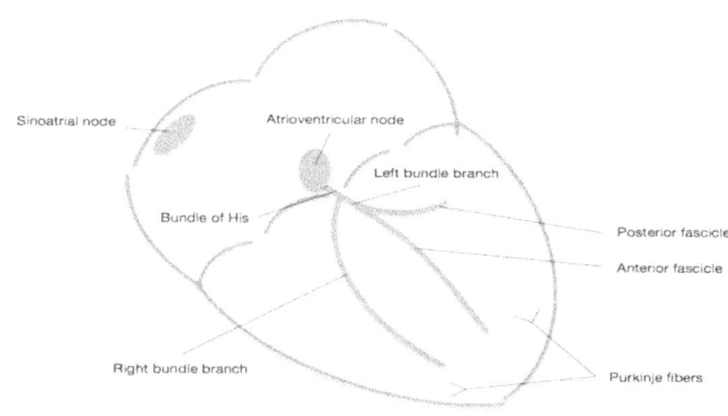

Step I: Evaluate ST segments and T waves.

Evaluate the ST segment for the presence of elevations or depressions, as well as abnormalities from the T wave. ST-elevation may indicate the presence of conditions such as acute myocardial injury, Prinzmetal's angina (variant), pericarditis, ventricular aneurysm, or myocardial ischemia.

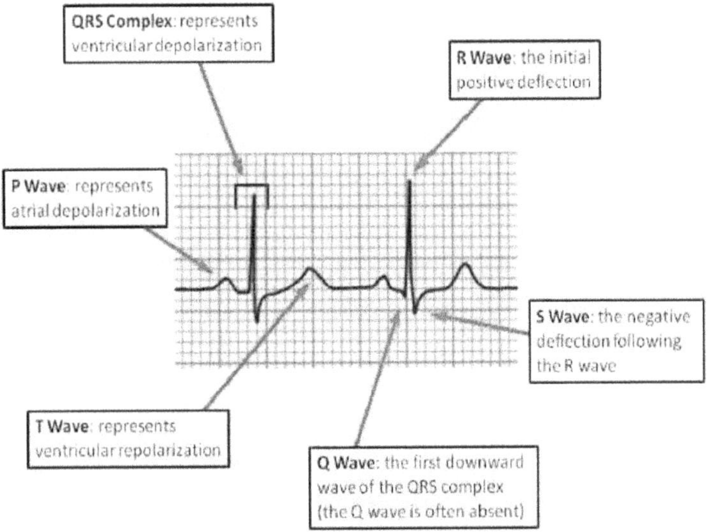

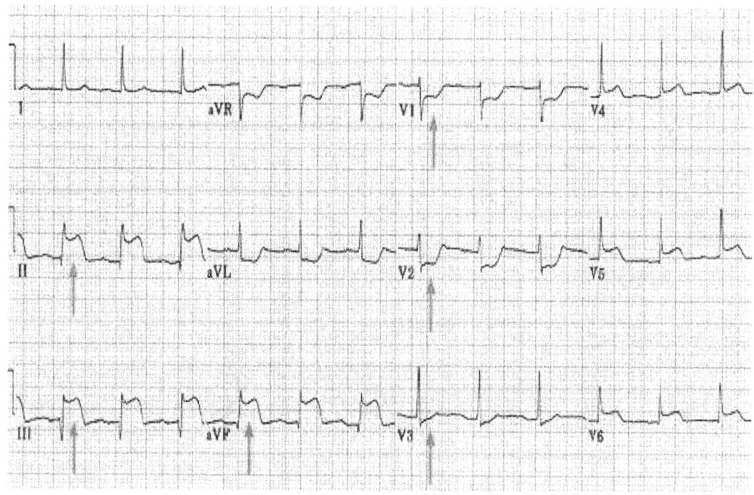

Step J: Measure the QT interval for specific diagnoses

The QT interval can be protected due to metabolic disturbances and pharmacological effects. It must be corrected for the heart rate as it is speed-dependent. The fixed QT interval is obtained by using the formula below:

Corrected QTI = (perceived QTI) / (square root of RR interval)

Corrected QTI is often reported with automated ECG interpretation.

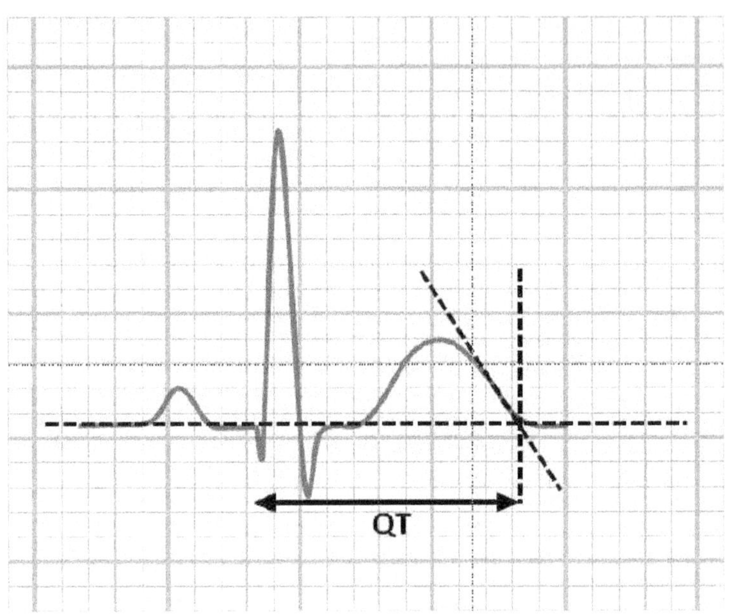

THE TYPES OF EKG

The American Heart Association does not recommend using EKGs to evaluate low-risk adults who are not showing symptoms. Doctors may suggest an EKG as a screening test if you have a family history of heart disease, even if you don't have any symptoms. If your symptoms come and go often, they may not be recorded during a standard EKG recording. In this scenario, your doctor may recommend remote or continuous ECG monitoring.

There are different kinds.

- **Holter monitor:** This is a small, portable device that records a continuous EKG, usually for 24 to 48 hours.
- **Event monitor:** This type is almost like a Holter monitor but only records a few seconds for a few minutes at a time. You usually press a button when you have symptoms.

WHAT HAPPENS DURING THE EKG PROCEDURE?

The EKG is a relatively simple test to perform. It's not invasive and doesn't hurt. It's placed on the skin to access the electrical impulses generated by the heart. An EKG machine records these pulses. The machine has four patches placed on the limbs; one is placed on each shoulder and one on each leg. These are called guide wires. Six patches (guidewire) are placed on the chest wall, starting just to the right of the sternum. The patches are placed in a semicircular shape that ends at the left armpit. These are called thoracic guides. These guidewires are connected to an EKG machine that records the tracks and prints them on paper.

Recent machines also have video screens that help the technician, nurse, or doctor decide whether the quality of the trace is adequate or whether the test should be repeated. EKG machines are also equipped with computer programs that can help interpret the EKG, although they are not entirely accurate.

In some situations, the doctor will want to view the heart from different angles after taking the first EKG. Then the chest cords can be attached to the right chest wall or back. The skin must be clean and dry to avoid electrical interference to obtain an acceptable trace for interpretation. Sometimes, that means shaving your chest hair or aggressively cleansing your skin. Chills or vibrations can disrupt the path and cause interference that affects the quality of the ECG trace. In general, the patient should remain still for 5 to 10 seconds without moving to obtain an accurate ECG.

WHY IS THIS BEING DONE?

An EKG provides two types of information. Firstly, by ascertaining the time intervals on the EKG, a physician can determine how long it takes for the wave to pass through the heart. Knowing how long it takes for a wave to travel from one part of the heart to the next shows whether the electrical activity is regular or irregular.

- To decipher abnormal heart rhythms that may have caused blood clots.
- Detect heart problems, including a recent or current heart attack, abnormal heart rhythms (arrhythmias), blocked coronary arteries, damaged parts of the heart muscle (due to a previous heart attack), an enlarged heart, and pericarditis.
- It detects non-cardiac conditions such as electrolyte imbalance and lung disease.

- To ascertain recovery from a heart attack, progression of heart disease, or the effectiveness of certain heart medications or a pacemaker.

GENERAL NOTES ON THE TECHNICAL ASPECTS OF THE ECG

For digital ECG programs that provide diagnostic interpretation, several technical aspects must be considered:

- Signal processing, including acquisition, conversion of analogue signals to digital signals, and filtering to remove noise (e.g., myopotentials, motion artifacts, baseline drift of respiration). Correct filtering is a critical step as it can significantly alter the final processed signal.
- In most automated systems, all ECG leads are now recorded simultaneously. The construction of representative model complexes (dominant complexes) with the exclusion of premature beats allows the formation of an average complex for each lead.

- Waveform recognition, with accurate determination of the start and offset of the different waves (P wave, QRS complex, T wave). Representative complex overlap and temporal alignment for each lead provides more accurate labelling of the wave start and offset Interval measurements (PR, QRS, and QT) and amplitude parameters. When performed, global range measurements are associated with higher values than single-lead measurements because they eliminate the isoelectric ranges present in each of the individual leads. This process is simple and straightforward when the ECG signal is recorded in normal sinus rhythm. However, it can become very complicated in the presence of atrial arrhythmias, which require temporal or spectral analysis for recognition and discrimination of fast atrial electrical activity.

Manufacturers' algorithms for determining wave initiation and motion vary, creating recurring differences in QRS duration and differences in QT interval measurements.

In a recent study, different current digital electrocardiographs were examined for their automatic measurement of RR, PR, QRS, and QT interval length on 600 ECGs. It included 200 ECGs during QT interval studies in normal subjects, 200 ECGs in normal subjects during maximal administration of moxifloxacin (known to slightly prolonging the QT interval), and 200 patients with genotyped variants of long QT syndrome. The measured intervals and durations show small but statistically significant group differences between manufacturers.

The absolute differences between the algorithms were comparable for QRS duration and QT interval in normal subjects but were significantly greater in patients with long QT syndrome. Deviations from the amplitude measurement have been reported less frequently, but the daily variability of the amplitude measurements has been described, leading to significant differences in the voltage measurements and, thus, in computer diagnostics.

Despite advances in the development of different algorithms, differences in measurement results remain, and the call for standardization and recommendations for wave definitions and references, launched as early as the 1970s, remains incomplete. Statements that use an accurate measure of ECG amplitudes and durations can bring experienced readers closer together in terms of sensitivity, specificity, and reproducibility.

However, explanations depending on the waveform configuration (e.g., repolarization) and the relationship between the waveforms (e.g., irregular P waves, atrioventricular conduction disturbances) may show little accuracy because the computer reading the EKG lacks the skills to recognise a human shape.

Interpretation using diagnostic algorithms in the treated ECG. These algorithms are proprietary and can function differently when applied to ECG signals processed by different methods. Measurement differences between different standard ECG systems can be large enough to change the diagnostic conclusions, which can have clinical consequences and, for example, interfere with the selection of candidates for cardiac resynchronization therapy, as QRS duration is the primary determinant of device implantation in these patients.

CHAPTER 2:
ECG/EKG TRACING

Parts of an EKG

The standard ECG has 12 leads. Six of the probes are considered "limb probes" because they are placed on the arms or legs of the individual. The other six wires are considered "precordial wires" because they are placed in the torso (precordium). The six limb leads are called leads I, II, III, aVL, aVR, and aVF. The letter "a" means "raised" because these leads are calculated as a combination of leads I, II, and III. The six precordial threads are V1, V2, V3, V4, V5, and V6 cables. Below is a typical 12-lead ECG waveform.

The Normal ECG

A normal ECG contains waves, intervals, segments, and a complex as defined below.

Wave: A positive or negative deviation from a baseline that indicates a specific electrical event. Waves on an ECG include P wave, Q wave, R wave, S wave, T wave, and U wave.

Interval: This refers to the timing between two specific ECG events. Frequently measured intervals on an EKG include the PR interval, QRS interval (also called QRS duration), QT interval, and RR interval.

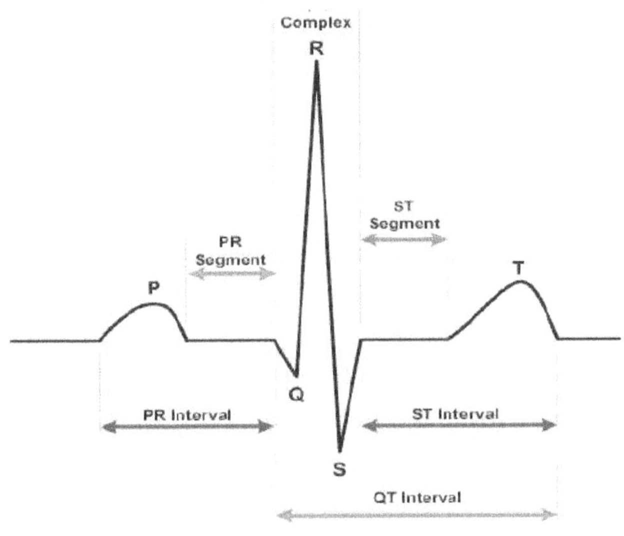

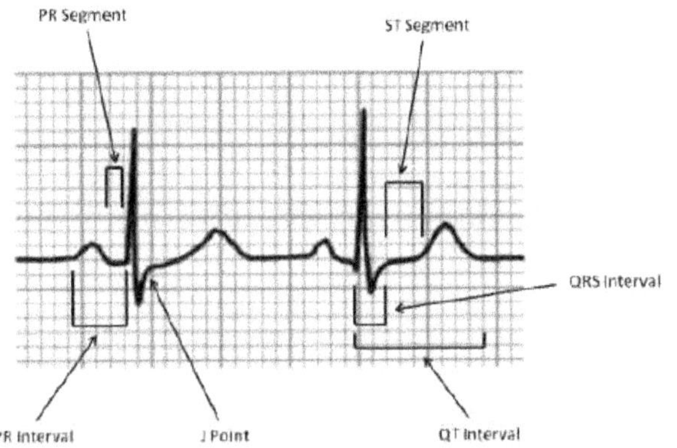

Segment - The length between two specific points on an EKG believed to be at baseline width (neither negative nor positive). The components of an ECG include the PR segment, the ST segment, and the TP segment.

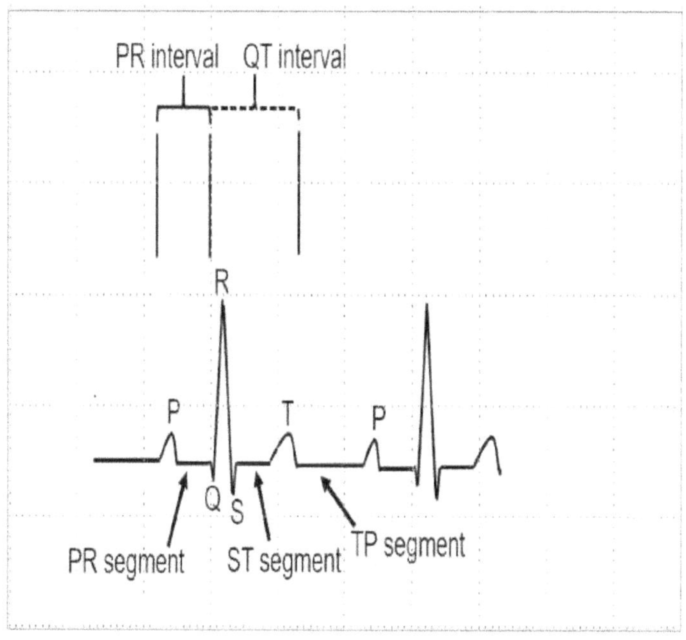

Complex: The combination of several grouped waves. The only essential complex on an EKG is the QRS complex.

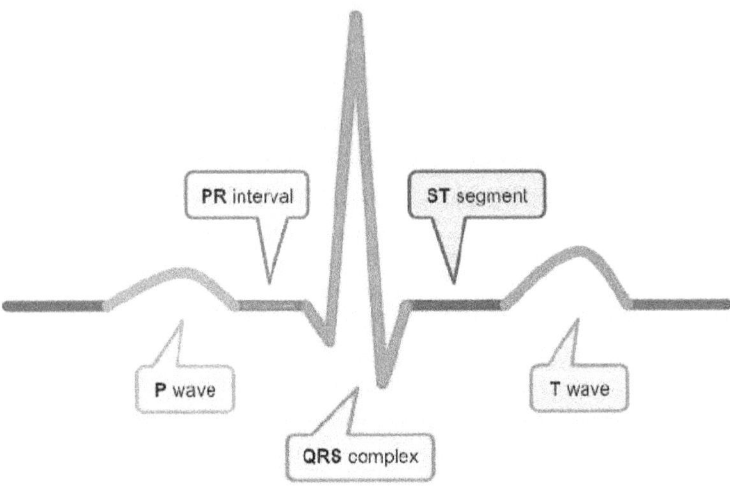

Point: The only point on an EKG is called the J point, where the QRS complex ends, and the ST segment begins.

Most of an EKG contains a P wave, a QRS complex, and a T wave. Each is explained separately in this tutorial, as well as each segment and interval.

The P wave indicates atrial depolarization. The QRS complex consists of a Q wave, an R wave, and an S wave and represents ventricular depolarization. The T wave appears after the QRS complex and indicates ventricular repolarization.

ALGORITHM PRECISION

The accuracy of the algorithm may vary depending on the manufacturer's automated program and the level of the boosters of the participating ballasts. In fact, these algorithms are generally tested against the diagnosis of expert physicians, cardiologists, electrophysiologists, or with the help of an expert consensus, considered the "gold standard." In addition, ECG interpretation is a mix of subjective and objective aspects, on which even cardiologists or experienced experts may disagree, resulting in significant interobserver variability. In addition, the ECG databases used to test software may not adequately represent the general population; in fact, they must be large and diverse enough to contain all possible clinical diagnoses that reflect everyday medical practice. A direct benchmarking of the performance of commercially available CIE programs has never been done, mainly due to the reluctance of manufacturers to have different algorithms.

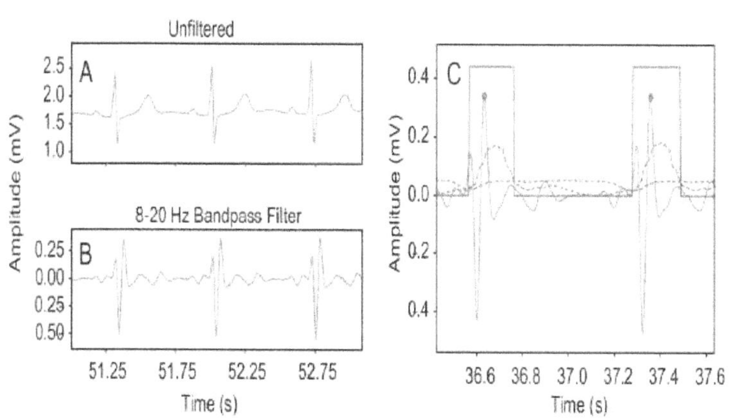

CONTRAINDICATIONS AND RISKS OF ECG/EKG

ECG/EKG is a safe test that does not cause any debilitation or complication to your health. There are no health conditions associated with an increased risk or adverse side effects from ECG.

LIMITATIONS OF ECG/EKG

The EKG or EKG machine is a potent and widely used screening tool for heart disease. It's relatively inexpensive, noninvasive, and easy to use. It has certain limitations. Understanding these boundaries is essential to put things in perspective. The ECG monitor displays the electrical activities generated by the heart and provides a picture of the cardiovascular rate and rhythm during the test. Heart defects can only occur intermittently, and the ECG must be taken at the "right" time to record episodes. At other times, a patient can have a completely normal EKG. For ease of things, many ECGs are taken while the patient is exercising, increasing the heart rate and putting pressure on the heart.

Stress ECG testing can reveal many hidden conditions in many situations that would otherwise go unnoticed.

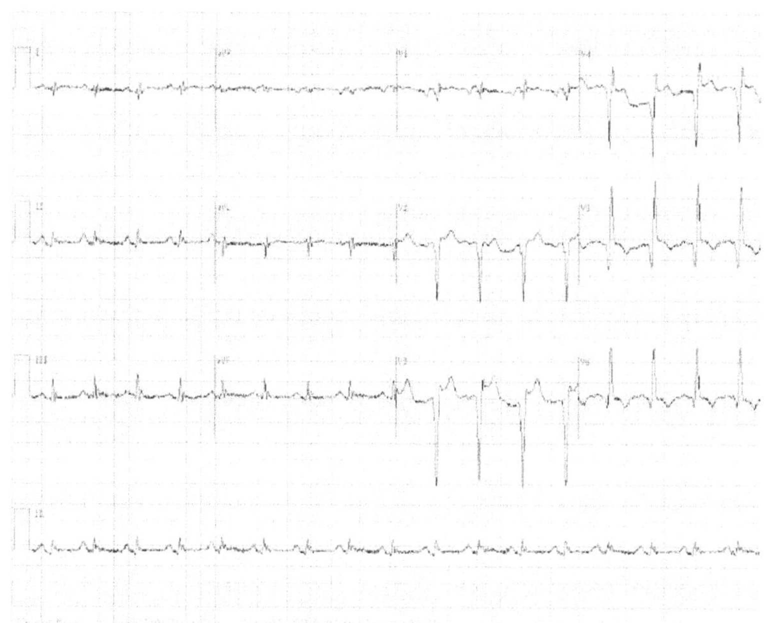

When the EKG machine shows an unusual pattern, there could be several independent reasons, including a standard variant. A doctor should do a more detailed examination, including other tests (e.g., Echocardiogram), to resolve the problem.

The false negative is probably the biggest concern with the EKG. For some heart patients, the EKG can be very normal, and yet their condition should be reflected on the EKG.

A precise EKG reading does not rule out that you have an underlying heart condition, and other symptoms, such as chest pain, should be considered, and further evaluation may be needed.

A good example is a fragile plaque (a form of atheroma). Vulnerable plaque is a rapidly growing deposit or degenerative build-up of lipid-containing plaque in the innermost layer of an artery wall. Because artery walls generally enlarge in response to plaque enlargement, they do not affect blood flow and cannot be detected even on a cardiac stress ECG test. Yet fragile plaque is one of the leading causes of a heart attack.

A stress ECG test requires high-quality stenosis to show a positive result as it is a good indicator of advanced heart disease; though, it is not the leading cause of a heart attack. The wrong diagnosis is common in clinical testing. A doctor must evaluate all tests before making a diagnosis.

The EKG is a static image and may not show any underlying severe heart problems when the patient has no symptoms. A common example of this is in a patient with a history of intermittent chest pain due to underlying severe coronary artery disease.

This patient can have a completely normal EKG at a time when he is not showing any symptoms. In such cases, the ECG recorded during an exercise test may reflect an underlying abnormality, while the ECG taken at rest may be normal.

Many abnormal patterns on an EKG can be nonspecific, meaning they can be seen under different conditions. They can even be a standard variant and show no deviations. Often a doctor can resolve these conditions with a detailed examination and sometimes with other heart tests (e.g., Echocardiogram, stress test).

In some cases, the EKG can be quite normal despite the presence of an underlying heart condition that would typically be reflected on the EKG. The reasons are mostly unknown, but it's important to remember that a normal EKG doesn't necessarily strike out the possibility of an underlying cardiac condition. In addition, a patient with cardiac symptoms may often require additional evaluations and tests.

THE ELECTRICAL CONDUCTION SYSTEM OF THE HEART

Coronary disease is the most common cause of death in developed countries, and patient deaths from cardiovascular disease increased by a third between 1990 and 2010

. This, along with a further expected increase in the prevalence of cardiovascular disease, has made the electrocardiogram (ECG) one of the most widely used instruments in clinical practice. To fully understand the EKG and interpret its results, it is necessary to understand the standard conduction system of the heart. The human heart contracts 2.5 billion times more than the person's average lifespan; this is achieved by the cardiac conduction system.

The electrical conduction system is a physiological system that stimulates the myocardium (heart muscle) to contract without external stimulation. The contraction of a cardiac myocyte (heart cell) is initiated by an electrical impulse (the heart pulse) that travels freely through the atrial and ventricular myocardium.

This phenomenon occurs because the myocytes of the heart are electrically coupled via so-called gap junctions. All myocytes in the heart have the ability to conduct a heart pulse; this implies that a single incitement of an atrial or ventricular myocyte can lead to contraction of the entire myocardium.

During normal activation of the heart, the heart impulse originates in the pacemaker cells of the sinoatrial (SA) node and spreads evenly through the atria. The heart pulse is then delivered to the atrioventricular (AV) node through the internodal pathways, where it travels through the conduction system of the ventricles and the ventricular myocardium. Irregularities in the standard cardiac conduction system can cause cardiac arrhythmias and, as such, an abnormal ECG. The heart cardiac conduction system is a network of cardiac muscle cells that process and send the electrical signal responsible for the coordinated contractions of each cardiac cycle. These special cells can generate an action potential themselves (self-excitation) and pass it on to other nearby cells (conduction), including cardiomyocytes. The components of the cardiac conduction system can be divided into segments that generate action potentials (knot tissue) and components that conduct them.

Although all parts have the capacity to generate action potentials and thus contractions of the heart, the sinus node (SA) is the main initiator and regulator of impulses in a healthy heart. This part makes the SA node the physiological pacemaker of the heart.

Other parts conduct the pulse sequentially from the SA node and then relay it to myocardial cells. When stimulated by the action potential, the myocardial cells contract in a synchronized manner, leading to what we call a heartbeat. The diffusion of electrical impulses and synchronous contraction of myocytes is facilitated by the presence of intermediate discs and gap junctions.

The heart's electrical conduction system causes the impulse generated in the sinus node (SA) to travel and stimulate the myocardium (heart muscle), causing it to contract. It consists of a coordinated stimulation of the myocardium that allows the execution of heart movements. The heart conduction system is responsible for the contraction of the heart muscle. Damage or erratic function of the cardiac conduction system can lead to severe and, in some cases, fatal clinical events. Any myocyte in the heart can contract when stimulated with the correct pulse. These impulses are generated by changes in the concentration of electrolytes inside and outside the pacemaker cells (a concentration gradient). The standard cardiac conduction system allows not only the generation of this impulse but also its automatic propagation through the atrial and ventricular myocardium, causing the heart muscle to contract fully.

WHAT IS THE HEART LIKE, AND HOW DOES IT WORK?

The human heart has four chambers, namely the right and left atrium and, therefore, the right and left ventricles. The right atrium and right ventricle of the heart collect blood from the body and pumps it to the lungs, while the left ventricle and left atrium receives blood from the lungs and pumps it to the body. Blood circulates in the body in the following ways:

Oxygenated blood from the lungs enters the left atrium through the vein called the pulmonary veins. The blood is pumped into the aorta via the left ventricle and distributed to the rest of the body. This blood supplies the organs and cells with oxygen and nutrients that are necessary for metabolism.

The blood returning to the heart is depleted of oxygen and contains the waste of metabolism, carbon dioxide. Blood is pumped to the right ventricle through the vena cava, which receives blood from the right atrium.

The right ventricle then transports blood via the pulmonary artery to the lungs, where carbon dioxide is removed, oxygen is replaced, and the cycle begins again.

Oxygen and nutrients needed by the heart are supplied by arteries that originate in the aorta. These blood vessels branch to provide oxygenated blood to all parts of the heart. The electrical impulse is generated in the upper chambers of the heart that initiates compression of the atria and pushes blood to the ventricles. There is a slight delay in filling the ventricles. The left and right ventricles then contract to pump blood to the body and lungs. The heart possesses an automatic pacemaker, called a sino-atrial node or SA, located in the right atrium. The SA node works independently of the brain to generate electricity to make the heartbeat.

Typically, the pulse generated by the SA node passes through the heart's electrical network and signals the atrial muscle cells to beat simultaneously, allowing for coordinated compression of the heart. The contraction of the atria pushes blood into the ventricles. The electrical signal generated at the pacemaker goes to a junction box between the atria and, therefore, the ventricles (the AV node), where it's delayed a couple of milliseconds for the ventricles to fill.

The contraction of these heart muscle cells is stimulated as a result of the electrical signal that travels through the ventricles. Ventricular contraction aids the pumping of blood to the body and the lungs (from the right ventricle). There is a short pause to allow the blood to return to the heart and refill before the electrical cycle repeats for the next beat.

CHAPTER 3: THE UNDERLYING PRINCIPLES OF HEART RHYTHM

ELECTROLYTES AND CONCENTRATION SCHEDULES

For a proper understanding of the electrical conduction system of the heart, it is essential to understand how cells work, especially the pacemaker and normal heart cells. The human body is made up of many cells, each of which is surrounded by a fat membrane and extracellular fluid and also contains all components of the cell electrolytes. The electrolyte concentration gradient, as well as the ability of electrolytes to cross the cell membrane, allow the generation of an electric current. For the contraction of a cardiac myocyte, the main electrolytes are sodium (Na), potassium (K), and calcium (Ca). Electrolytes enter and exit the cell through two main routes: tiny pumps built into the cell membrane and ion channels in the cell membrane. The sodium-potassium pump plays a vital role in this process by pushing sodium out of the cell and pumping potassium into the cell.

A concentration gradient arises because the pump continuously pumps potassium into the cell, resulting in a higher concentration of potassium inside the cell than outside, resulting in a change in the intracellular potential.

In this process, the opposite happens for sodium because a higher sodium concentration is created outside the cell with a lower sodium concentration inside. The other method by which electrolytes enter and exit cardiac myocytes are through ion channels. Unlike the sodium-potassium pump, which passes multiple electrolytes, ion channels are specific to a single electrolyte. Ion channels are voltage-dependent and allow each specific electrolyte to enter or exit the cell, depending on the concentration gradient of that specific ion. When potassium channels are open, potassium leaves the cell; when sodium channels open, sodium enters the cell. It is these opposite reactions that create an electrical charge across the cell membrane. Therefore, it is the principle encompassing the generation of the heart pulse.

DEPOLARIZATION AND REPOLARIZATION

Contraction and subsequent relaxation of the heart are achieved by depolarization and repolarization of all cardiac myocytes. Change in the porosity of the cell membrane directly affects the concentration of electrolytes in and around the cell, creating a pulse. This heart impulse spreads through the surrounding tissue causing depolarization of the entire myocardium. Depolarization involves an increase in electrical current across the cell membrane, forcing a change in the resting potential of cells and generating an action potential that propagates through the heart. Repolarization, in simple terms, is the process of returning the cell to its normal restive state.

ECG and electrical activity of the myocardium

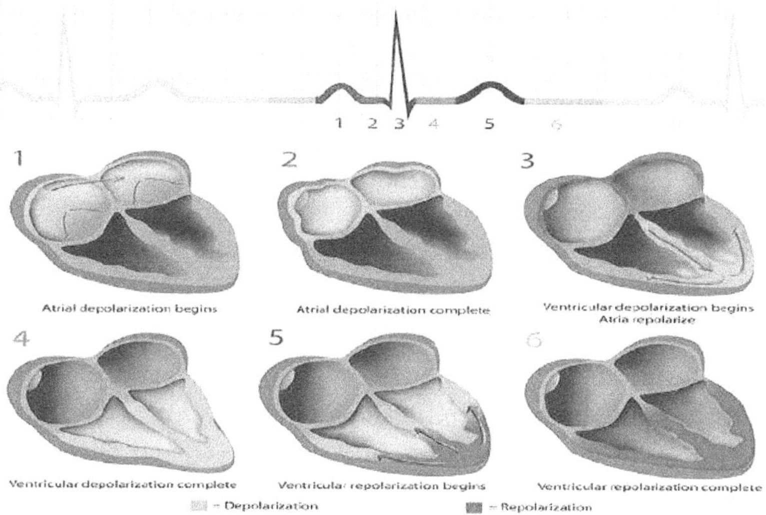

ACTION POTENTIAL OF A CARDIAC MYOCYTE

This refers to a quick change in voltage across the cell membrane of a muscle or nerve cell when proper stimulation is applied. A cardiac action potential is described in five main stages (0-4). Stage four represents the resting cell; currently, the cell has a potential of about -90mV11. An electric current of a surrounding pacemaker cell or myocyte (muscle cell) stimulates the membrane opening of the sodium and potassium pump to allow sodium to enter, causing the cell potential from negative (-90 mV) to positive (20 mV).

This is called phase 0 and is commonly referred to as the depolarization phase. So open calcium channels through which calcium can enter the cell, causing a slight dip (phase 1) and stabilisation of the cellular potential (plateau phase, phase 2) around ten mV and closes the sodium channel. Then calcium is released from intracellular stores—an increase in calcium concentration in the cell and causes contraction.

In the post-contraction phase 3, the calcium channels close, and the potassium close open channels that cause the cell to repolarise and return to its resting potential from 90mV 10. The cardiac myocyte quickly spreads from cell to cell once it experiences an action potential. However, once a cell becomes depolarised, it becomes insensitive for a short time; it means that the cell can only be stimulated more to reach its resting state. There are two phases in the refractory period:

- The absolute refractory phase in which no stimulation of any magnitude causes the cell to contract; and the relative refractory phase in which a sufficiently large electric current causes the cell to contract. This prevents an excessively rapid contraction of a heart muscle cell and results in a stable and continuous propagation of electrical current through the myocardium.

ACTION POTENTIAL OF A PACEMAKER CELL

Pacemaker cells, unlike cardiac myocytes, coordinate the rhythm and rhythm of the heartbeat and, as such, have automaticity. Pacemaker cells are responsible for generating the heart pulse and therefore have a different action potential than standard cardiac myocytes. Pacemaker cells do not really contract and, as such, do not have a plateau phase in their action potential. The action potentials of pacemaker cells are different from those of normal cardiac myocytes in that the automatic cells have the ability to initiate an electrical current or pulse without any external stimulation. In comparison, a normal cardiac myocyte can contract only when stimulated by an external impulse from an electrically coupled cell. Ion currents play a crucial role in the functioning of pacemaker cells. After Repolarization, the potassium ions create an outlet stream. This is followed by an incoming stream of sodium ions. These sodium ions are activated upon repolarization and are followed by a slow incoming flow of calcium ions that are activated upon depolarization of the cell membrane. Pacemaker cells are crucial for a contraction of the heart and are found in three areas: the SA node, the bundle of the His, and the AV node.

However, the cells found in these areas are classified as automatic; the rate of depolarization varies between the three types of automatic cells, the SA node depolarization phase (phase 4) and, therefore, the fastest rate of fire - approximately 60 to 100 times per minute. The AV junction has a slower pace of fire of 40 to 60 times per minute and finally branches, and Purkinje fibers bundle at a rate of fire of fewer than 40 times per minute; therefore, the design is not competitive.

CHAPTER 4: SINUATRIAL NODE

The most important aspect of heart contraction is the cardiac conduction system. The conduction system allows an electrical impulse generated by the pacemaker cells in the SA node to travel efficiently through the atrial and ventricular myocardium, causing constant and timely contraction of the heart muscle. The heart electrical conduction system is made of the SA node, the AV node, the bundle His, the bundles of braces, and the Purkinje network. The heart rate comes from the SA node in the right upper atrium and has primary responsibility for the electrical activity of the heart. The inaugural node (SA node) is a flat, elliptical collection of specialized knot tissue measuring up to 25 millimeters (mm) in length. The lump is situated in the superior posteromedial wall of the right atrium close to the aperture of the superior vena cava, which is indicated by the terminal sulcus (the junction of the venous sinus and the right atrium). Here it is found in the subepicardial layer of the heart, often covered with a relatively thin layer of fat.

In the center, the SA node is filled with pale staining cells called pacemaker cells (P). Cytologically, P cells contain a very large central nucleus but a small number of other organelles (possibly the cause of the pale staining). Unlike the surrounding heart muscle cells, P cells have very few cytoplasmic myofibrils and no Sarcotubular apparatus.

The P cell population begins to decrease towards the periphery of the SA node, where other transition cells become more apparent. These thin spindle cells look like a cross between the mentioned P cells and typical cardiomyocytes. These transition cells form bridges between the P cells and the neighboring atrial cells.

The pacemaker receives its blood supply from the sinus node branch of the arteria coronaria. In about 60% of people, this artery may be a branch of the proper coronary artery (so in the remaining 40%, it comes from the left coronary artery). There are numerous autonomic ganglion cells lining the anterior and posterior SA nodes. However, none of these nodes seems to end in the pacemaker cells. Instead, P cells contain cholinergic and adrenergic receptors to respond to neurotransmitters released by surrounding autonomic ganglion cells.

INTERNODAL CONDUCTION PATH

The internodal conduction pathways are part of the intra-atrial conduction network. In addition to traveling through the right atrium, these pathways provide direct points of communication between the sinoatrial and atrioventricular nodes. The internodal conduction path is divided into anterior, middle, and posterior branches.

The anterior internodal pathway stems from the anterior margin of the SA node. It continues forward and runs around the superior vena cava, where it releases the Bachmann bundle. The anterior internodal band runs anteroinferior to the atrioventricular (AV) node, entering the node through its superior margin.

The middle internodal path originates from the superior posterior margin of the SA node. It continues behind the superior vena cava to the edge of the interatrial septum. The path rotates caudally in the interatrial septum to enter the AV node through its superior margin. Finally, the posterior internodal route emerges from the posterior border of the sinus node. It follows a posterior course around the superior vena cava and passes through the crista terminalis to the Eustachian crest (valve of the inferior vena cava). The route then enters the interatrial to the AV node through the posterior surface.

These conduction pathways transfer the action potential slightly faster than the surrounding cardiomyocytes. They contain Purkinje-like cells (deficient in myofibrils), which ensure that the action potential reaches the AV node at the right time. The blood supply to these pathways is comparable to the blood supply to the right atrium, the diacritic branch of the left coronary artery.

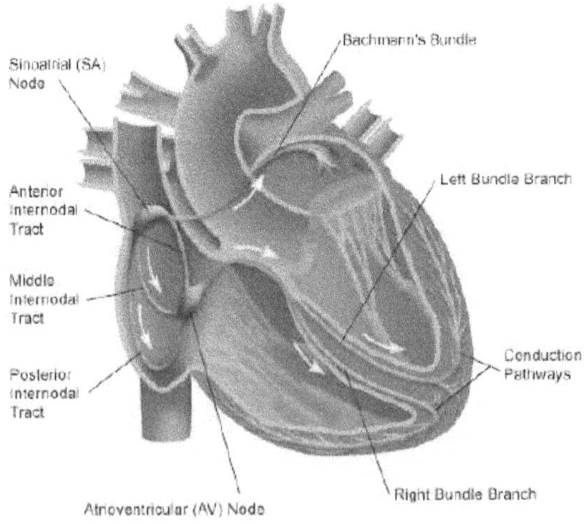

INTERATRIAL CONDUCTION PATHWAY

It is also called the Bachmann bundle, which refers to a preferred path of special cardiomyocytes that enhance the conduction of impulses between the atria. The path branches from the anterior internodal path to the level of the superior vena cava. The Bachmann bundle passes through the interatrial groove (an external landmark of the interatrial septum) and passes through the limbus of the fossa oval. A path of adipose tissue separates the Bachmann bundle from the limbus. The trail branches into right and left branches that go to the right and left atria, respectively. The right branch can be divided into the upper and lower arm. The upper arm originates from the external junction of the superior vena cava and the atrium (near the location of the SA node). The forearm opens into the entryway of the right atrium. The left branch gives some structural support to the anterior atrial wall and continues to envelop the left atrium. Almost the top part of the left branch passes in front of the openings of the left pulmonary veins. The lower portion extends caudally to the vestibule of the left atrium.

Histologically, the interatrial conduction path is a series of parallel myocardial strands that move through the subepicardial layer. Bachmann bundle myocytes are enclosed in thin septa made up of tightly packed collagen fibrils. This continuous shell also forms interseptal connections (the function of which is not yet clear).

Five types of cells in the interatrial tract are:

Cells rich in myofibrils, which are the same as normal cardiomyocytes.

Myofibril-poor cells: resemble Purkinje cells; they are numerous in the course.

P cells, such as those described in the sinus node.

Thin transition cells: short and narrow.

Wide transition cells - Longer and wider than thin transition cells.

The presence of these specialized cells facilitates the rapid conduction of the action potential through the left atrium, minimizing the depolarization delay between the atria. The Bachmann bundle receives its blood supply from the sinus node branch of the coronary artery.

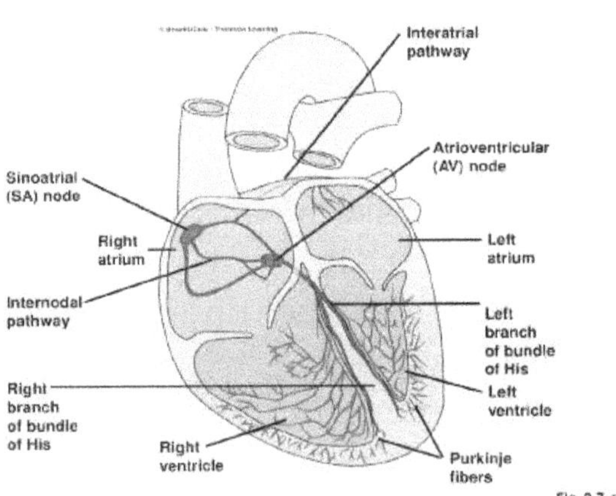

CHAPTER 5: ATRIOVENTRICULAR NODE (AV)

It is another specialized structure in the heart, like the SA node described above, which also aids in the conduction of impulses. It is often referred to as the secondary pacemaker of the heart. Under normal circumstances, it functions as a conductor of electrical activity from the SA node to the ventricles of the heart. This is the only pathway by which the action potential can travel from the atria to the ventricles; because the atrioventricular septum consists of a cartilage structure that cannot conduct electrical impulses. The AV node is located in the inferior posterior portion of the interatrial septum and is smaller than the SA node.

More precisely, the node rests on the triangle of the atrioventricular node (Koch's triangle or Koch's triangle). This triangle is surrounded by the coronary sinus (basal), the septal petal of the tricuspid valve (inferior), and the tendon of the inferior pyramidal space (inferior vena cava tendon or Todaro's tendon) (superior). The semi-oval node occupies the subendocardial layer in the Koch triangle. The top of the node extends anteroinferior.

It crosses the fibrous skeleton of the heart and forms the first part of the atrioventricular (AV) bundle (of His). The histological composition of the AV node is relatively similar to that of the SA node. The main discrepancies are fewer P cells and more transition cells than that of the SA node.

The AV node accepts arterial blood from the branch of the atrioventricular node. It arises from the inferior interventricular branch of the right coronary artery in 80% of individuals. In the remaining 20% of individuals, the branch of the atrioventricular node originates from the diacritic branch of the left coronary artery. There is also a remarkable number of autonomous ganglion cells around the AV node (as seen in the SA node). However, none of these is synapse with the AV node. Like the cells of the SA node, the cells of the AV node also have adrenergic and cholinergic receptors to respond to autonomic stimuli.

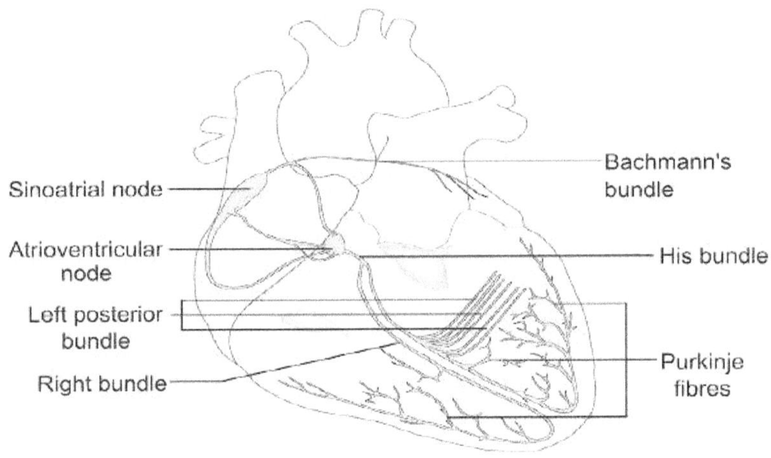

THE ATRIOVENTRICULAR (AV) BUNDLE

The atrioventricular bundle is the initial segment of the AV node that enters the membranous portion of the interventricular septum through the fibrous trigone. In cross-section at the fibrous body, the AV bundle may appear oval, quadrangular, or triangular. A unique and essential feature of the AV package is that it allows only the "forward" movement of action potentials. Hence, the retrograde transmission of electrical impulses from the ventricles to the atria is not possible in a normally functioning heart. The AV bundle is delivered by the anterior and inferior interventricular branches of the coronary arteries.

RIGHT AND LEFT BUNDLE BRANCHES

As the tubercle travels from the membranous septum to the muscular interventricular septum, it branches into the right and left bundles. The crus dextran, which is Latin for the right bundle branch, emerges from the AV bundle to the membranous interventricular septum. It is around a group of narrow beams that travel through the myocardium before moving superficially in the space of the subendocardial layer. It goes to the right side of the interventricular septum, where it branches off the ventricular walls before moving to the ventricular apex. Here, it enters the Septomarginal moderator band (swept marginal band) before reaching the anterior papillary muscles. The terminal arborization of the right branch innervate the papillary muscle and re-innervate the rest of the ventricular wall.

The left bundle branch or crus sistrum (Latin) branches from the atrioventricular bundle to the beginning of the muscular interventricular septum consists of many small bundles that turn into flattened leaves. These bundles occupy the left half of the muscular ventricular septum. The blade moves in the subendocardial space as it advances towards the ventricular apex. Here triples in the rear, septal and anterior divisions. The branches will continue to activate the anterior and posterior papillary muscles, the interventricular septum, and the left ventricle walls.

PURKINJE FIBERS

The bundles are populated with subendocardial branches called Purkinje fibers. These cells are often much larger than those of the encompassing heart muscles and perform very differently from cells within the anterior AV node. The subendocardial branches are found along the entire length of both bundles in the subendocardial layer. They spread to the top of the heart and then meander up and back through the walls of the ventricles. The fibers have many more gap junctions than the AV button cells and the surrounding myocytes. As a result, they can transmit impulses six times faster than ventricular muscles and 150 times faster than AV node fibers. The more significant number of gap junctions allows more ions to travel from one cell to another, increasing the conduction velocity. There are also fewer myofibrils in Purkinje cells, which results in little contraction (i.e., shorter or absent refractory periods) in these cells. Therefore, the beams can achieve near-instantaneous transmission of the action potential to the rest of the ventricle as soon as it passes through the AV node.

This augments for the delay within the atrioventricular node and permits the ventricles to shorten briefly after the atria.

Take note that the main branches of the atrioventricular bundle are isolated by connective tissue sheaths. This prevents premature excitation of the adjacent heart tissue. As a result, the papillary muscles will depolarise first, followed by the ventricular apex and then the walls. The depolarization pattern also extends from the endocardium to the epicardium as the fibers are located in the subendocardial layer.

CHAPTER 6: PHYSIOLOGY OF SA AND AV NODES

SINUATRIAL NODE

They have a reduced resting membrane potential than surrounding heart muscle cells and transition cells because heart muscle cells have a particular ability to stimulate themselves (self-excitation or automatism). The onset of the action potential depends on the ion channels that allow the passage of ions in and out of cells. Cardiomyocytes have fast-acting sodium ion channels (Na +), slow sodium-calcium ions (Na + -Ca2 +), and slow/fast potassium ions (K +) (among other important channels that control ion balance). This automatism affects, in particular, the below indices:

- There is a huge concentration of extracellular Na + outside the NODES fibers.
- A relatively large number of Na + channels are already open.
- There is passive Na + diffusion in P cells between heartbeats through "leaky" sodium channels.
- The slow influx of sodium causes a slow increase in the membrane potential of the cell, gradually moving it closer to the threshold to generate an action potential.

Therefore, the heart P cells in the SA node depolarise more easily than other heart cells. The SA node is also closely connected to the surrounding heart muscles through the internodal and interatrial conduction pathways. Therefore, the generated action potential can be quickly transferred to other cells. This allows the SA node to set the rate at which the heart cells depolarise and then contract, making it the pacemaker of the heart. On average, the SA node can generate between 60 and 100 beats per minute at rest.

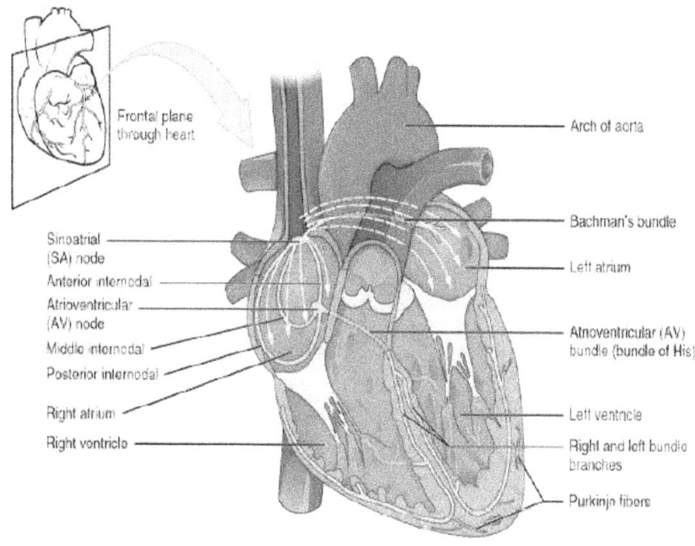

Anterior view of frontal section

ATRIOVENTRICULAR NODE

While the main function of the AV node is to facilitate the journey of the depolarization wave to the ventricles, it also has extra functions. Without a functioning SA node, the AV node can act as a pacemaker for the heart. Remember, it also has P cells capable of establishing a rhythm (albeit slower) (45 to 60 beats per minute). The AV node is also responsible for the deceleration of the passage of the electrical impulse going to the ventricles. This important phenomenon gives the ventricles more time to rest and fill with blood from the contractile atria. An important characteristic of transitional cells and P cells in the AV node is that they have less closely spaced nodes in the intermediate disks. Therefore, there is more resistance to driving in this part of the tramline than in other areas.

IMPULSE GENERATION AND CONDUCTION

Now let's summarise it all and describe the stages of cardiac conduction:

The SA node generates the action potential.

The action potential crosses the internodal and interatrial conduction pathways and causes atrial systole.

The pulse reaches the AV node and is delayed to facilitate ventricular filling (ventricular diastole).

The pulse then travels from the AV node to the AV bundle.

It then spreads through the bundle branches and subendocardial tissue and causes ventricular systole.

The entire cardiac conduction system is affected by the autonomic pathway. The sympathetic stimulation of the conductive tissue comes from the cardiac plexus, while the parasympathetic influence comes from the vagus nerve (CN X).

Activation of the nervous system leads to divulge of adrenaline (epinephrine) and other adrenergic neurochemicals. They bind to beta one and beta two receptors found in SA and AV junctions, as well as along supportive conduction pathways.

The general impact of the sympathetic system is an increase in the SA node depolarization rate. Hence, it increases the general heart rate (increased chronotropic). Since these adrenergic receptors are also present in heart muscle cells, the sympathetic impulse will act on these cells, increasing the contractile force (increased inotropy). Therefore, overall cardiac output will increase.

On the opposite hand, the parasympathetic activation of muscarinic receptors within the SA and AV nodes will have the other effect as compared to the sympathetic system. Parasympathetic stimulation slows down activation of the SA node, slowing the heart rate. It also decreases cardiomyocyte contractility, effectively reducing cardiac output. Any abnormality in the conduction path, whether congenital or acquired, can cause an abnormal rhythm or arrhythmia. Arrhythmia implies that the heart is not beating the way it should be at the right time. These can take the form of a heartbeat that is too fast (tachycardia) or too slow (bradycardia).

There may also be abnormal sites that generate an electrical pulse (ectopic beats). Arrhythmias, as well as a physiological electrical current through the heart, can be tracked by an electrocardiogram (EKG or ECG). While some rhythm irregularities are transient and may go unnoticed, others can cause life-threatening changes in cardiac output.

CHAPTER 7:
RHYTHM AND HEART RATE

Electrodes on the chest wall can detect electrical impulses generated by the heart. Different leads provide numerous electrical images of the heart. By interpreting the trace, the doctor can learn more about heart rate and rhythm, as well as blood flow to the ventricles (indirectly).

The rate refers to how fast your heart is beating. Typically, the SA node generates an electrical pulse of 50 to 100 times per minute. Bradycardia (bradycardia = slow + cardia = heart) describes a heart rate of less than 50 beats per minute. Tachycardia (tachycardia = fast + cardia = heart) describes a heart rate of more than 100 beats per minute.

Rhythm refers to the type of heartbeat. Typically, the heartbeat in sinus rhythm and any electrical impulse generated by the SA node causes a ventricular contraction or heartbeat.

There are several irregular electrical rhythms, some are normal, and some are potentially dangerous. Some electrical rhythms do not generate a heartbeat and cause sudden death.

Rhythms strip with a standard 12-lead ECG. Examples of heart rhythms are:

- A normal sinus rhythm
- Sinus tachycardia
- Sinus bradycardia
- Atrial fibrillation
- Atrial flutter
- Ventricular tachycardia
- Ventricular fibrillation

There may also be retards in the transmission of the electrical impulse in any part of the system, including the SA node, atria, AV node, or ventricles. Some abnormal impulses cause normal heart rate fluctuations, and others can be life-threatening. Some examples are:

- First degree AV block
- Second degree AV block, type I (Wenckebach)
- Second degree AV block, type II
- Third-degree AV block or complete heart block
- Right bundle branch block
- Left bundle branch block

There may also be shorts that can lead to abnormal electrical pathways in the heart that result in abnormalities in speed and rhythm.

Wolfe-Parkinson-White (WPW) syndrome is a condition in which an abnormal accessory pathway in the AV node can cause tachycardia.

A sinus rhythm

Sinus rhythm is regular with average deviations and intervals P, Q-R-S, T. Speed = 60-100 at rest.

Sinus bradycardia

This is a rhythm at a rate of less than 60 per minute in an adult.

Sinus tachycardia

Sinus tachycardia is a rhythm at a rate greater than 100 per minute in an adult.

First-degree heart block

First-degree heart block (Adam Stokes) sinus rhythm is sinus rhythm with an extended PR interval> 0.20 seconds thanks to delayed transmission from the atria to the ventricles.

Second degree AV heart block

A second-degree AV block is generally classified as Mobitz Type I (Wenckebach) or "Mobitz Type II." Mobitz type I is characterized by progressive lengthening of the PR interval until a QRS complex is exited.

A Mobitz type II is characterized by an intermittent, interrupted QRS that's not during a Mobitz Type II cartridge. Mobitz Type II block should be evaluated because it's a block that will rapidly evolve into a full Adams-Stokes syndrome.

Third-degree heart blocks

It is referred to as a complete heart block, which is a rhythm where there is no relationship between P and QRS waves, respectively. In this scenario, the P to P intervals are regular but not related to the QRS complexes on the ECG.

Supraventricular tachycardia

Supraventricular tachycardia (SVT) is a fast atrial rhythm with narrow QRS complexes when the pulse originates above the bundle branches (above the ventricles).

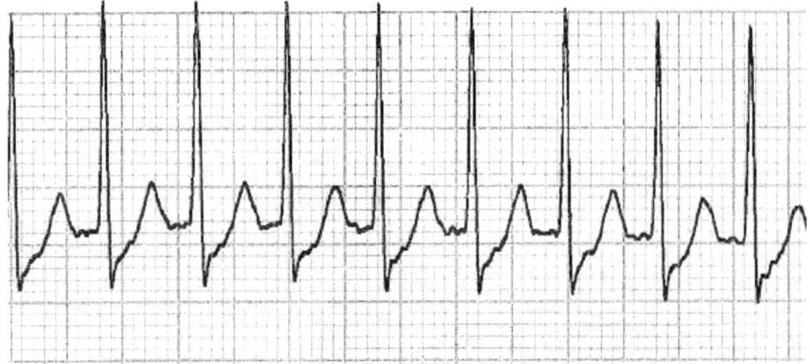

Atrial fibrillation

Atrial fibrillation is a prevalent arrhythmia. This rhythm is characterized by the absence of waves in front of the QRS complex and a very irregular heartbeat.

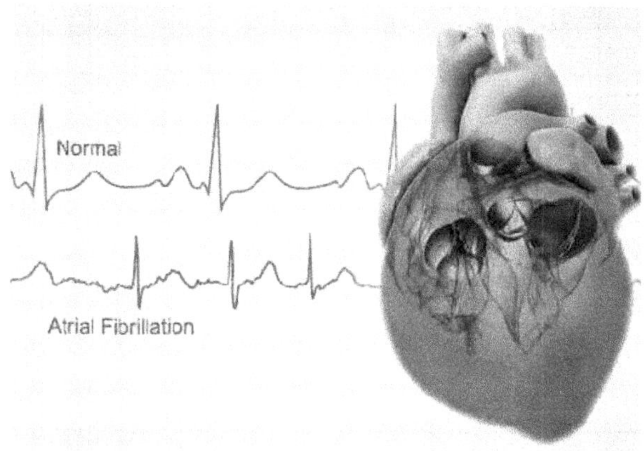

Atrial flutter

Atrial flutter is a supraventricular arrhythmia characterized by a "sawtooth" flutter on the ECG that represents multiple P waves for each QRS complex.

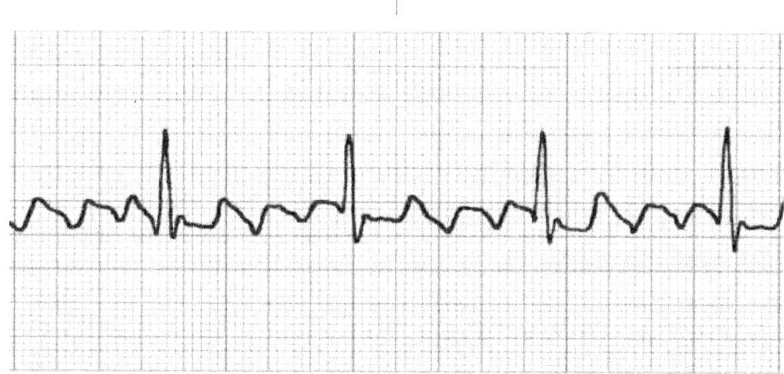

Asystole

Asystole is also known as the "flatline," in which no electrical activity can be seen on the heart monitor. Not responsive to electrical defibrillation.

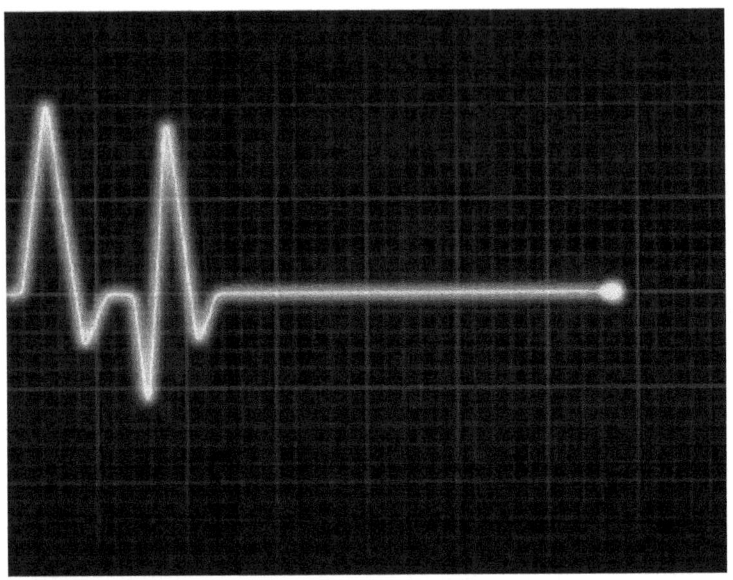

Pulseless Electrical Activity

It can be almost any organized EKG rhythm in an unresponsive patient and has no palpable pulse. Therefore, a PEA rhythm cannot be learned. However, it should not be misconstrued with the specific heart rate scenarios listed above.

Ventricular tachycardia; Ventricular tachycardia (V-tach or VT) is characterized by strangely enlarged QRS complexes, absence of P waves, and usually a rate greater than 100 per minute. It can swiftly degenerate into ventricular fibrillation and death.

Ventricular fibrillation; This is abbreviated as Vfib or VF. It is identified by a chaotic wave pattern coupled with the absence of a pulse. VF can be sensitive to electrical defibrillation.

The ECG trace can also provide information about whether the cells of the heart muscle are conducting electricity properly. By describing the shape of the electrical waves, an anesthesiologist can determine if the blood flow to parts of the heart muscle is decreasing. The presence of an acute block associated with myocardial infarction or a heart attack can also be determined. This is the main reason why an EKG is taken as soon as possible if a patient has chest pain.

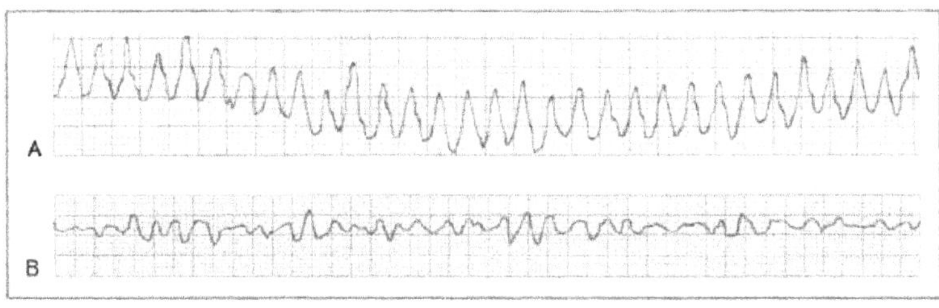

How to Analyze The Rhythm & Rate: Steps to reading an EKG/ECG

How do you know whether to act immediately or wait for a consultation with an expert? Below are some points to help you better understand what you are seeing.

1. EVALUATE YOUR PATIENT

It must come first! There are many clues you can learn from taking the EKG that will help you analyze and act on what you see.

- Is the patient's skin warm, dry, wet, or sticky?
- What is your color?
- Do they have chest pain?
- Do you feel the peripheral impulses?
- Is your patient talking to you or having trouble catching his breath?
- What is your hair charging?
- Do they have underlying heart problems?
- What is your basic physical activity?
- Have you ever had an EKG?

First degree AV block

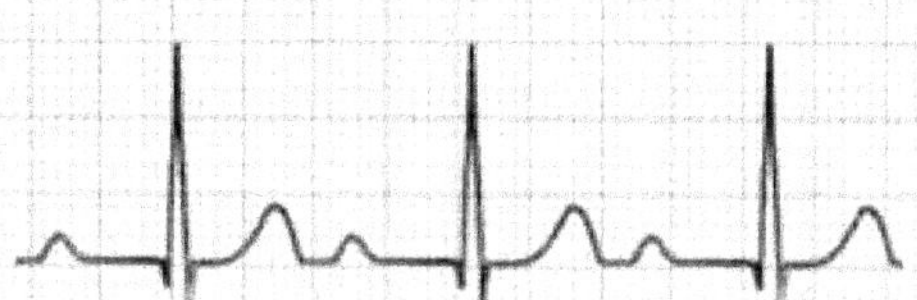

Second degree AV block (Mobitz I or Wenckebach)

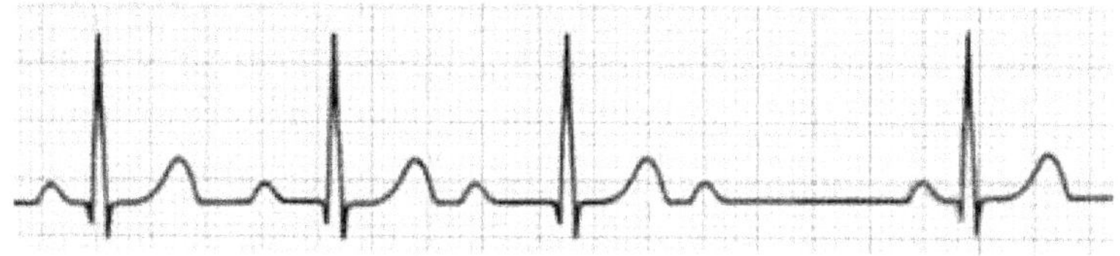

Second degree AV block (Mobitz II)

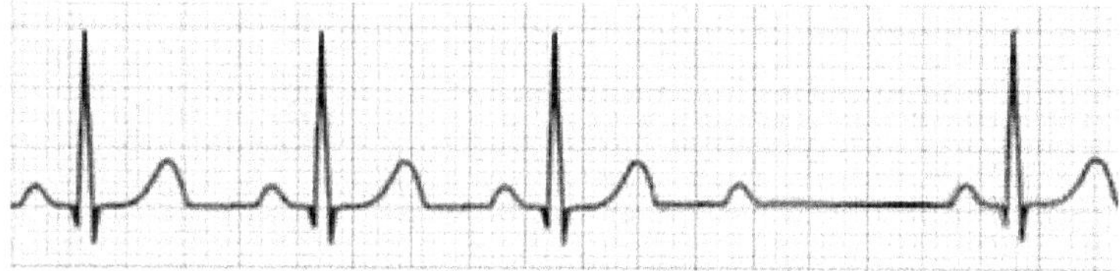

Second degree AV block (2:1 block)

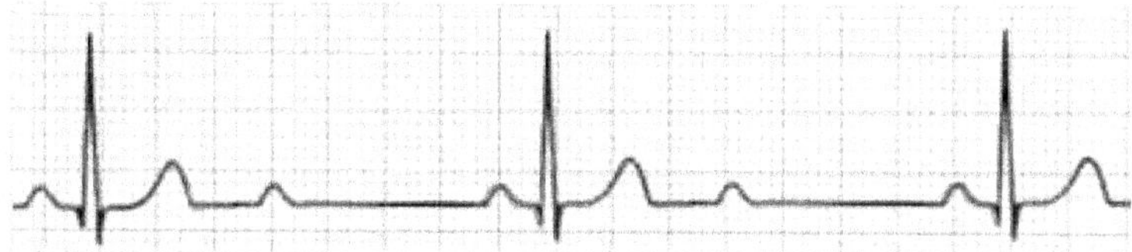

Third degree AV block with junctional escape

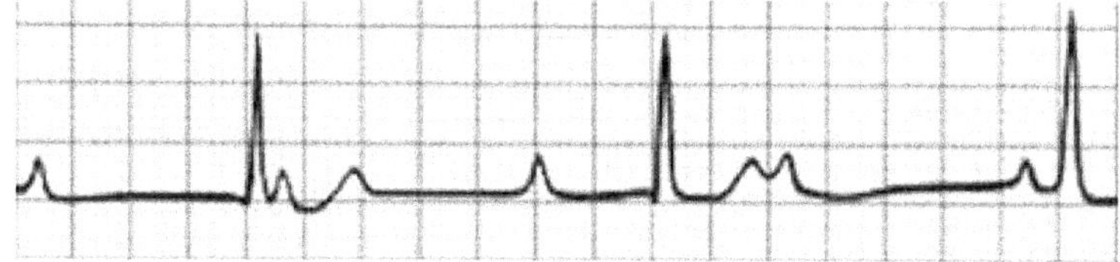

Mere Looking at a sheet of paper does not provide enough information. A heart rate of 38 may be expected for an athlete. But it may also require immediate pacemaker placement if accompanied by chest pain, shortness of breath, and an EKG interpretation of a third-degree heart block.

2. KNOW YOUR NORMALS

Don't worry about all the intricate details when reading and interpreting EKGs. A normal heart rhythm consists of a P wave, QRS, and T wave. Knowing the average amplitude, deviation, and duration of each segment is essential for accurate interpretation of the rhythm and ECG.

Amplitude: Measures the voltage of the beat and is determined by the height of the wave, measured by each square vertically on the graph. 10mm= 1 mv.5 squares = 0.5 mV and 2.5 squares = 0.25 mV

Duration: How long it measures, measured by horizontal squares

- Average heart rate for an adult:
- Normal = 60 to 100 bpm
- Tachycardia> 100 bpm
- Bradycardia <60 bpm

We can calculate the bpm by dividing 1500 by the number of SMALL squares between two R waves intervals.

We can ascertain bpm by dividing 300 by the number of BIG squares between two R waves.

REGULAR rhythms

The rate equals 300 / number of LARGE squares between consecutive R waves.

VERY FAST rhythms:

The rate equals 1500 / number of SMALL squares between consecutive R waves.

SLOW or IRREGULAR rhythms:

Rate = number of waves R X 6

The number of complexes (counting R waves) in the rhythm band gives the average cadence over ten-second timing. This is multiplied by six, which equals 1 minute to get the average beats per minute (bpm)

3. DETERMINE YOUR RHYTHM

Check the EKG to see if the frequency is regular and how fast the heart is beating; both are important to rhythm performance. The speed at which a tempo is pushed can help determine the stability of the tempo. A stable rhythm is often attributed to a normal patient with a stable rhythm. Slow or fast can be a good or bad sign depending on the patient's presentation and the associated rhythm. The speed is usually determined by the electrical circuitry that "drives" the heart. Rhythms performed above the atria are generally over 60 and tend to be abnormal when the rhythm is fast (atrial flutter, atrial fibrillation, supraventricular tachycardia). Rhythms performed under the atria are slower and tend to be unstable when the rhythm is irregular (heart blocks).

One more note on the rate: know what medications your patient is on. Many heart drugs have beta-adrenergic effects that correlate with a slower heart rate, such as beta-blockers. It is essential to determine whether the heartbeat is regular or irregular. A regular heartbeat has all the aspects discussed above.

Irregular rhythms can include:

- Regularly irregular (i.e., a recurring pattern of irregularities)
- Irregularly irregular (i.e., completely disorganized)

To ascertain if a rhythm is regular, mark out several consecutive R-R intervals on a piece of paper and then move them along the rhythm band to ensure the following intervals are equal.

UNDERSTANDING YOUR HEART RATE BY THE NUMBERS

Standard Heart Rates in Children:

Newborn: 110 – 170 bpm

Two years: 85 – 125 bpm

Four years: 75 – 115 bpm

Six years+: 60 – 100 bpm

You can measure your heart rate. First, determine your heart rate by placing a finger on the radial artery close to the wrist. Then sum up the number of beats per minute at rest.

Other areas in your body where your heart rate can be measured are your neck (carotid artery), groin (femoral artery), and feet (dorsalis pedis and posterior tibial arteries).

Below are key numbers to keep in mind:

• An adult's resting heart rate is usually between 60 to 100 bpm

• Sportsmen or people on certain medications may have a lower average resting rate.

• The average heart rate for children 1 to 12 years old is one of 6 possible underlying causes of bradycardia

A full medical evaluation is needed to determine the cause of a slow heart rate. An electrocardiogram (EKG or EKG), laboratory tests, and other diagnostic studies may be performed.

- Possible medical causes of a slow heart rate are:
- Irregular or abnormal heart rhythms
- A congestive cardiomyopathy
- Chronic side effects from medications
- stroke
- an electrolyte imbalance
- sinus disease
- hypothyroidism
- injury to the atrioventricular (AV) node

The average heart rate for babies 1 to 12 months old is 110 to 170 beats per minute.

4. IDENTIFY DEADLY RHYTHMS

When assessing lethal rhythms on a 12-lead electrocardiogram, it's important to remember that rhythm alone can be fatal, as well as what the EKG shows in terms of heart function. A bad-smelling rhythm can quickly lead to impending heart failure if left untreated. Some dangerous heart rhythms are:

- Mobitz Type II (type 2 heart block)
- Third-degree heart block
- Ventricular tachycardia
- Idioventricular rhythms

Other heart rhythms that may be of concern include:

- Atrial fibrillation
- Atrial flutter
- Nodal recurrent atrioventricular tachycardia (AVNRT)
- Re-entering atrioventricular tachycardia (AVRT)
- Ectopic atrial rhythms
- First degree atrioventricular (AV) block
- Union rhythms
- Multifocal atrial tachycardia (MAT)
- Second degree atrioventricular (AV) block type I
- Second-degree atrioventricular block type II E.
- Third-degree atrioventricular (AV) block
- Ventricular Tachycardia (VT)

- Roaming Atrial Stimulator (WAP)
- Bifascicular block
- Left anterior fascicular block (LAFB)
- Left atrial magnification (LAE)
- Left bundle branch block (LBBB)
- Left posterior fascicular block (LPFB)
- Left ventricular hypertrophy (LVH)
- Poor R wave progression
- Right atrial magnification (RAE)
- Right bundle branch block (RBBB)
- Right ventricular hypertrophy (RVH)
- Trifascular block

CHAPTER 8: ARRHYTHMIA

Heart rate is a measure of heart activity. A slow heart rate is considered to be less than 60 beats per minute for an adult or a resting child. Your heart rate should be strong and stable without missing a heartbeat. If it beats more slowly than usual, it could indicate a medical problem.

An arrhythmia, also known as cardiac dysrhythmia, cardiac arrhythmia, heart arrhythmia, or irregular heartbeat, is an irregularity with the rate or rhythm of a person's heartbeat. When an arrhythmia occurs, the heart could beat too fast, beat very slowly, or even beat with an irregular rhythm. It is called tachycardia when the heartbeats faster than normal. And when it beats too slow, the condition is called bradycardia.

Arrhythmia is caused when there are changes in heart tissue, activity, or changes in electrical signals which are responsible for controlling the heartbeat. These changes can be due to damage from disease, symptoms, genetics, or an injury. This can cause a person to faint or have difficulty in breathing. An electrocardiogram remains the most common test in diagnosing an arrhythmia.

In such cases, the doctor can introduce the placement of a device that will correct the irregular heartbeat, offer the solution of a surgery which will repair the tissues overstimulating the heart, or he might simply recommend medicines. But how exactly are arrhythmias identified?

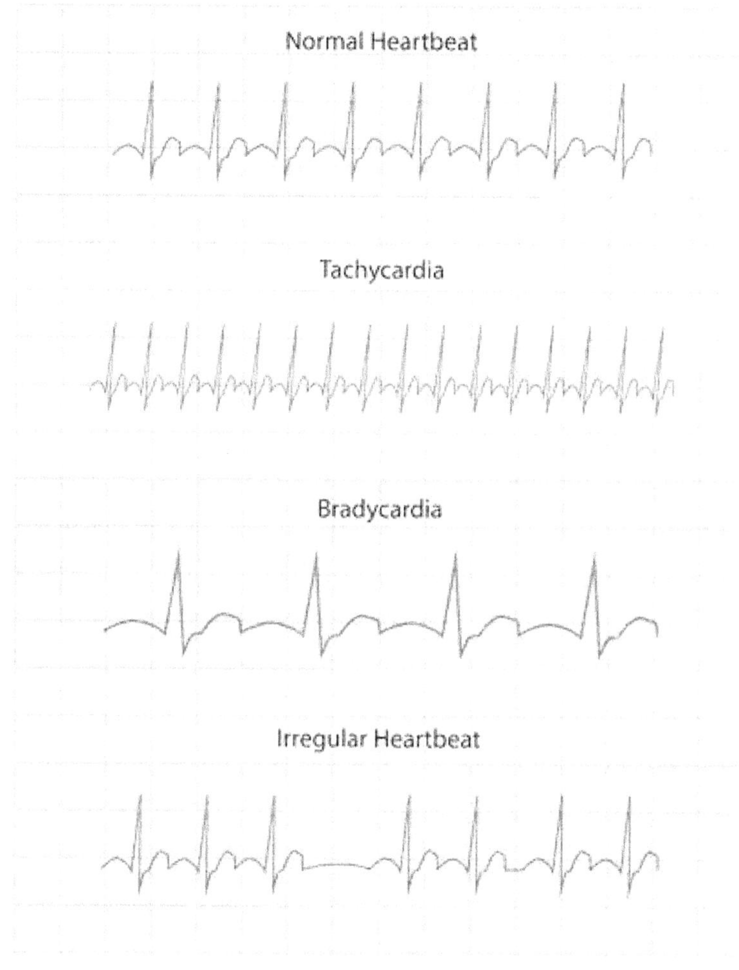

They are identified by where they come or originate from in the heart. They are also recognized by whether they cause the heart to increase in speed or decrease.

The treatment for cardiac arrhythmia can either eliminate these irregular heartbeats or simply controlled. But it is important that one adopts a healthy heart lifestyle because some worse cases of arrhythmias are often caused when the heart is weak or damaged.

If there's an abnormal heartbeat, what then is an abnormal one? Every human heart is made up of four chambers; The upper chambers and the lower chambers. The rhythm of the heart is controlled by the sinus node in the right atrium. This mode produces electrical impulses which start each heartbeat. When these pulses are produced, the atria muscles contract, causing blood to be pumped into the ventricles.

These electrical impulses now become a cluster of cells which are called the atrioventricular (AV) node. The AV node then slows down the electrical signal before it is sent to the ventricles. Due to this slight delay, the ventricles have time to be filled with blood. The muscles of the ventricles contract when electrical impulses reach them, then blood is pumped to the lungs and other body parts.

This process goes smoothly in a healthy heart, but when it is slightly or drastically changed, arrhythmias arise.

In most cases, a slow heart rate is an indication of an extremely healthy heart. For example, athletes often have a lower resting heart rate than usual because their hearts are healthy, and they don't have to work as hard to pump blood around the body.

However, if a slower heart rate is accompanied by other symptoms, it could be a sign of something more serious. Arrhythmia describes an irregular heartbeat. With this condition, a person's heart can beat too fast, too slow, too fast, or with an asymmetrical rhythm. It occurs when the electrical signals that coordinate the heartbeat don't work correctly. An irregular heartbeat can resemble a heartbeat or a beating heart.

Many cardiac arrhythmias are harmless. However, if they occur as a result of a weak or damaged heart, arrhythmias can lead to severe and life-threatening symptoms and complications.

Some arrhythmias can cause problems with heart chamber contractions due to:

- Do not allow the lower chambers (ventricles) to fill with enough blood, as an abnormal electrical signal causes your heart to pump too fast or too slow.
- As an abnormal electrical signal, not getting enough blood into your body is causing your heart to pump too slowly or irregularly.
- Do not allow the upper chambers (atria) to function correctly.

An arrhythmia sets in when there is a problem with the electrical system that controls the average heart rate. A faulty electrical system can cause your heart to beat too fast, too slow, or irregularly.

Types of Arrhythmias

1. Tachycardia: This is when the heartbeat is fast, i.e., greater than a hundred (100) beats per minute.

2. Bradycardia: This is when the heartbeat is slow, i.e., heart rate is less than sixty (60) beats per minute.

However, not every tachycardia or bradycardia necessarily signals a heart disease. Just like the heartbeat tends to increase after an exercise or decrease when a person is asleep.

Tachycardias that originate in the atria include:

a. Atrial fibrillation. This is a rapid heart rate, which is a result of chaotic electrical impulses in the atria. These signals cause rapid, uncoordinated, and weak contractions of the atria.

The chaotic electrical signals bombard the AV node, and when this happens, it results in an irregular or rhythm of the ventricles. Atrial fibrillation may occur temporarily, but some episodes do not end easily, except if treated. Serious complications like stroke could be associated with atrial fibrillation.

b. Atrial flutter: This is quite similar to atrial fibrillation. Except those heartbeats in atrial flutter are usually more organized, with more rhythmic electrical impulses than it is in atrial fibrillation. Atrial flutter may also lead to serious complications like stroke.

c. Supraventricular tachycardia: This is an expansive term that includes many forms of arrhythmia that originate above the ventricles in the atria or AV node. These types of arrhythmia cause sudden episodes of palpitations that start and end unexpectedly.

d. Wolff-Parkinson-White syndrome: This is a type of supraventricular tachycardia, where there is a presence of an extra electrical pathway between the atria and the ventricles at birth. This pathway gives way for electrical signals to pass through the atria and ventricles without passing through the AV node. Hence, causing short circuits and fast heartbeat. But the symptoms of this syndrome may not be experienced till one becomes an adult.

Tachycardias that originate in the ventricles include:

a. Ventricular tachycardia: This is a rapid, regular heart rate that arises from the abnormal electrical signals in the ventricles. The rapid heart rate prevents the ventricles from filling and contracting enough to pump blood efficiently throughout the body. If one has a healthy heart, then ventricular tachycardia may not result in any complications. But for individuals with weak and unhealthy hearts, prompt medical treatment is required. However, if the heart is not restored to a normal condition in the next few minutes, the results might be fatal.

b. Ventricular fibrillation: This occurs when rapid, turbid electrical impulses cause the ventricles, rather than pumping blood to the body, to vibrate ineffectively. Like ventricular tachycardia, this could also be fatal if not attended to in a few minutes.

Most times, people who experience ventricular tachycardia are those who have either experienced trauma or have underlying heart disease.

c. Long QT syndrome: This syndrome is a heart disorder that comes along with an increased risk of fast, turbid heartbeats. The fast heartbeats caused by changes in the electrical system of the heart may result in fainting or could be life-threatening in worse cases.

On the other hand, if an individual has a slow heart rate, or the heart is not pumping enough blood, then they might have one of these types of bradycardia;

a. **Sick sinus syndrome**. If the sinus node is not sending impulses properly, your heart rate may alternate between bradycardia and tachycardia. Sick sinus syndrome can also arise due to scarring near the sinus node, which slows down or blocks the travel of impulses. This syndrome is most common in adults.

b. **Conduction block**: This is a block of the heart's electrical pathways, which either occurs near the AV node or in the AV node that lies between the atria and the ventricles.

The impulses between the halves of the heart may be slowed down or blocked. It is all determined by the location and type of block. Some blocks may result in no signs or symptoms, while others may lead to skipped beats or bradycardia.

c. **Premature heartbeats**: Most people do not know this, but a premature heartbeat is an extra beat, although it feels like a skipped beat. One can have a premature beat once in a while, so it rarely signifies a serious problem.

At the same time, a premature heartbeat is capable of causing long-term arrhythmia, especially with people who are suffering from heart diseases. However, when premature heartbeats are recurrent (lasting for several years), it weakens the heart.

Premature heartbeats can occur when you are resting or could be due to stress, use of stimulants, or carrying out strenuous tasks.

RISK FACTORS FOR ARRHYTHMIA

Many risk factors can militate against your heart's electrical system and therefore cause arrhythmias. Caffeine, alcohol, tobacco, illegal drugs, diet drugs, certain herbs, and even prescription drugs can cause arrhythmia. Medical issues, such as high blood pressure, coronary heart disease, and diabetes, contribute to the development of arrhythmias. Arrhythmias become more familiar with age.

SYMPTOMS OF ARRHYTHMIA

Arrhythmias may not necessarily lead to any signs or symptoms. In fact, a doctor might find that a patient has an arrhythmia even before the patient does. Also, noticeable signs and symptoms do not mean you have a serious problem.

However, the effects on the body are usually the same if the heart rate is too fast, too slow, or too irregular.

Some of the symptoms of arrhythmias include:

- Palpitations (feeling of irregular or floating heartbeat)
- The weakness and tiredness
- low blood pressure
- Dizziness
- Heart failure
- Collapse and cardiac arrest
- Difficulty feeding (in babies)
- Chest Pain
- Sweating
- Lightheadedness
- Anxiety
- Shortness of breath
- Fainting
- A fluttering feeling in the chest

The symptoms of arrhythmias can resemble other conditions. Always consult your doctor for a diagnosis. How are arrhythmias diagnosed?

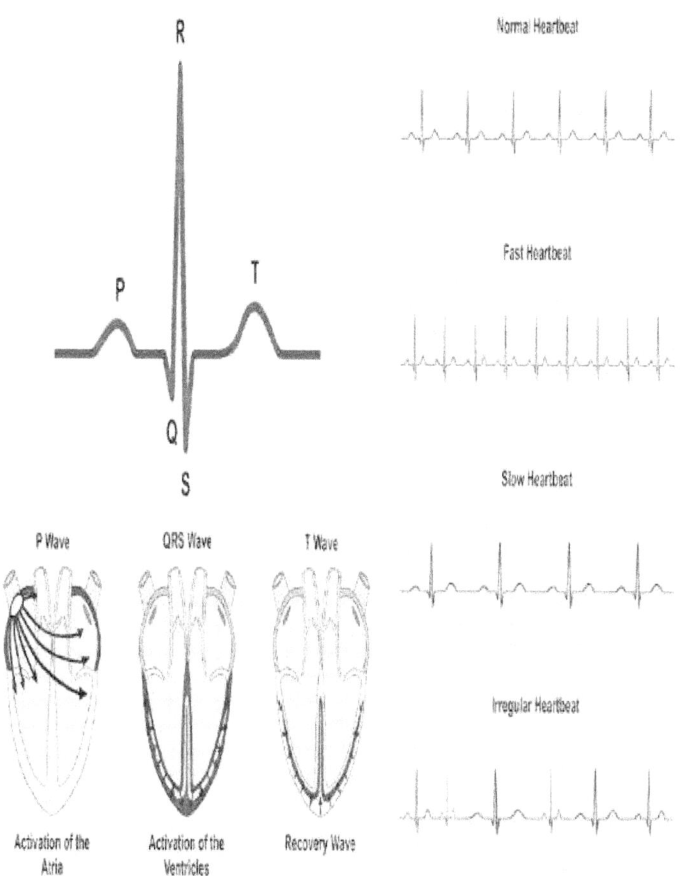
Normal and Abnormal Heart Rate
R
P
T
Q
S
P Wave
QRS Wave
T Wave
Activation of the Atria
Activation of the Ventricles
Recovery Wave
Normal Heartbeat
Fast Heartbeat
Slow Heartbeat
Irregular Heartbeat

Some of the tests that can be used to diagnose arrhythmias are:

Electrocardiogram (ECG) An EKG is a measure of your heart's electrical activity. Putting electrodes at specific locations on your body creates a graphical representation or trace of electrical activity while an EKG machine receives and interprets electrical activity. An ECG shows the presence of arrhythmias, heart damage caused by ischemia or myocardial infarction (heart attack), a problem with one or more heart valves, or something similar. There are several variants of the ECG test:

- **ECG AT REST**. For this procedure, clothing is removed from the upper body, and small sticky pieces called electrodes are put on a specific part of the body like on the chest, arms, and legs. These electrodes are connected with cables to the EKG machine. The EKG machine starts and records your heart's electrical activity for about a minute, and you have to lie down during this EKG.
- **EXERCISE ECG OR STRESS TEST**. It is connected to the ECG machine, as described above. However, rather than lying, exercise by walking on a treadmill or pedaling on a stationary bike while recording the EKG. This test is done to ascertain changes in the EKG during exercise.

- **AVERAGE ECG SIGNAL.** This procedure is going in the same way as a resting EKG, except it records your heart's electrical activity over a more extended period of time, usually 15 to 20 minutes. Signal averaged ECGs are performed when an arrhythmia is suspected but are not visible on a resting ECG. The mean signal ECG has a higher sensitivity to an abnormal ventricular activity called "late potentials." Signal averaged ECG is used and rarely used in clinical practice.
- **ELECTROPHYSIOLOGICAL STUDIES (EPS).** A nonsurgical but minimally test in which a catheter is inserted into a large blood vessel in your leg or arm and advanced towards your heart. This allows your doctor to find the origin of the arrhythmia in the heart tissue. Then your doctor can determine how best to cure it. Most of the time, your doctor can treat the arrhythmia by eliminating it during the examination.
- **HOLTER MONITOR**. A continuous ECG recording is taken over a period of 24 hours or longer. The electrodes are played on the chest and connected to a small portable ECG recorder using lead wires. Holter monitoring can be performed when an arrhythmia is suspected but is not visible on a resting ECG.

Arrhythmias can be transient and may not appear during the shorter resting ECG recording times. You perform your daily activities except those where you sweat excessively. This can cause the electrodes to loosen or fall during the procedure. These activities include showering.

- **EVENT MONITOR.** This is just like a Holter monitor, except it only starts recording the EKG when you feel symptoms. Event monitors generally take longer than Holter monitors.
- **MOBILE HEART MONITORING.** This is comparable to a Holter monitor and event monitor. The EKG is continuously monitored to help detect arrhythmias, which are recorded and sent to your doctor whether or not you have symptoms. You can also start checking in if you have symptoms. These monitors can be used for up to 30 days.
- **IMPLANTABLE LOOP RECORDER**. This is a miniature cardiac recording device that is implanted under the skin that covers your heart. It can record the heart rate for up to 2 years and is useful for diagnosing intermittent or rare arrhythmias.

HOW IS AN ARRHYTHMIA TREATED?

Some arrhythmias can cause little or no problems. In that case, you may not need treatment. When an arrhythmia is causing symptoms, you have several treatment alternatives. The physician will prescribe a treatment based on the type of arrhythmia you have, the severity of your symptoms, and whether you have other conditions, such as diabetes, kidney failure, or heart failure.

- **Lifestyle:** caffeine, stress, and alcohol can cause cardiac arrhythmias. It is advised to avoid caffeine, alcohol, or anything else that could be causing the problem. If your health care provider believes that stress is a cause, he may recommend meditation, stress management classes, an exercise program, or psychotherapy to relieve stress.
- **Medicine:** Medicines are available to treat arrhythmias. Your doctor will recommend medications based on the type of arrhythmia you have, if you have other health conditions, or if you are taking other medications.
- **Cardioversion:** In this procedure, the doctor sends an electric shock to your heart through your chest. This will stop some very fast arrhythmias such as atrial fibrillation, supraventricular tachycardia, or atrial flutter. It is connected to an EKG monitor, which is also connected to the defibrillator.

The electric shock is delivered during the ECG cycle to change the rhythm to a normal rhythm.

- **Ablation**: it is a **slightly** invasive but nonsurgical procedure performed in the electrophysiology lab. The physician inserts a tiny flexible tube called a catheter into your heart through a vessel in your groin or arm. The healthcare provider will use a method such as radiofrequency ablation to destroy the arrhythmia site. The procedure uses very high-frequency radio waves to heat tissue until the area is destroyed. Cryoablation is another procedure used. For this, an ultra-cold substance is placed on the arrhythmia site to freezes the tissue and destroys the site.
- **Pacemaker:** a small tool placed under the skin, often in the chest, just below the collarbone. Sends electrical signals to start or control a slow heart rate. A permanent pacemaker can be used to set the heartbeat if the heart's natural pacemaker (the SA node) is not working correctly or if its electrical pathways are blocked.
- **Implantable Cardioverter Defibrillator (ICD):** This is a little device that resembles a pacemaker. It is placed under the skin, often just below the collarbone. An ICD detects the rhythm of your heartbeat.

When your heart rate exceeds the level entered into the device, an electric shock is sent to the heart. This corrects the rhythm to a slower, average heart rate. ICDs are used to send an electrical signal to normalize a slow heart rate, and they are used for fast, life-threatening arrhythmias such as ventricular tachycardia or ventricular fibrillation.

- **Surgery:** Surgery is usually only done when all other treatments have failed. Surgical removal is a major operation that requires general anesthesia. The surgeon bisects your chest to reach your heart and destroys or removes the tissue causing the arrhythmia.

COMPLICATIONS OF AN ARRHYTHMIA

Some arrhythmias have no complications. However, more severe arrhythmias can lead to heart failure, stroke, or even cardiac arrest.

Living with an arrhythmia includes lifestyle changes like avoiding caffeine, alcohol, or other triggers and taking medications as directed. It may also include the insertion of a pacemaker or implantable cardioverter-defibrillator. If you are using a pacemaker or implantable cardioverter-defibrillator, ask your doctor about any restrictions or lifestyle changes you may need to practice or work on. Working with your doctor can promote your health and wellness.

Key points about arrhythmias

- Arrhythmia is an irregular heart rhythm.
- It can occur in the sinus node, the atria, or the atrioventricular node.
- Some arrhythmias cause little or no problems.
- Other arrhythmias can lead to severe complications such as heart failure, stroke, or even cardiac arrest.
- Many treatment options are available to treat arrhythmias, including drugs, devices, cardiac ablation, and surgery. Many arrhythmias can be cured with procedures.

https://www.webmd.com/heart-disease/atrial-fibrillation/heart-disease-abnormal-heart-rhythm

https://my.clevelandclinic.org/health/diseases/16749-arrhythmia

https://en.m.wikipedia.org/wiki/Arrhythmia

CHAPTER 9: ARRHYTHMIAS OF THE SINOATRIAL (SA) NODE

This is the inability of the natural pacemaker (sinus node) to get a pulse that suits the body's needs. It causes irregular heart rhythms (arrhythmias). Sick sinus syndrome is also referred to as sinus node dysfunction or sinus node disease, a neighborhood of specialized cells within the upper right chamber of the heart. This zone controls your pulse. Naturally, the sinus node creates a constant rhythm of electrical impulses; the pace changes based on your activity, emotions, rest, and other factors. Furthermore, the term sick sinus syndrome is applied to the clinical syndrome and includes chronic NS dysfunction, often depressed escape pacemakers, and atrioventricular node conduction disorders. The term sinoatrial disease is used side by side with sick sinus syndrome and describes a range of abnormalities that can lead to deep sinus bradycardia, sinus pauses, sinus arrest, sinoatrial node exit block, and chronotropic incompetence, defined as responding inappropriately to demands—physiological stress during exercise.

In sick sinus syndrome, electrical signals are abnormally stimulated. The rate may be irregular, interrupted by long pauses or an alternating combination of these rhythm problems. Sick sinus syndrome is relatively rare, but the risk of developing it increases with age.

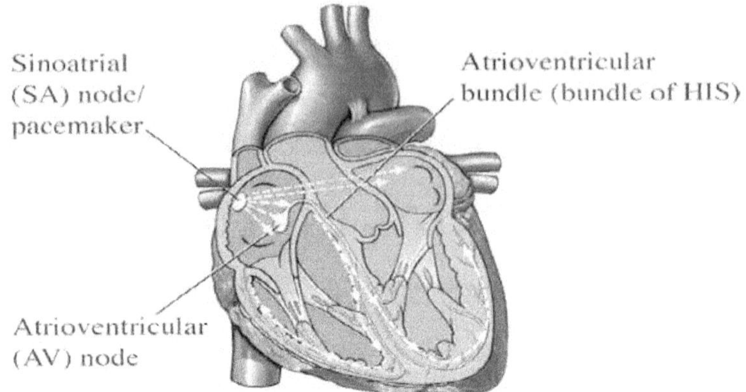

SYMPTOMS ARRHYTHMIAS OF THE SINOATRIAL (SA) NODE

A good percentage of people with sick sinus syndrome have few or no symptoms. The symptoms can be mild or come and go, making them difficult to spot at first.

Signs and symptoms of sick sinus syndrome can include:

- fatigue
- Dizziness or vertigo
- Fainting or nearly fainting
- Breathing problems
- Chest pain or discomfort
- Confusion
- Slower than average heart rate (bradycardia)
- Feeling of fast and floating heartbeat (palpitations).

CAUSES ARRHYTHMIAS OF THE SINOATRIAL (SA) NODE

Your heart is formed from four chambers: two upper chambers (atria) and two lower chambers (ventricles). The rhythm of your heart is generally controlled by the sinus node, a neighborhood of specialized cells within the upper right section of the heart (atrium). This natural stimulator produces electrical signals that activate each beat of the heart. From the sinus node, electrical signals travel through the atria to the ventricles, leading to contraction and pumping of blood to the lungs and body.

If you've got sick sinus syndrome, your sinus node isn't working correctly, leading to a heartbeat that's too slow (bradycardia), too fast (tachycardia), or irregular. Problems with the sinus node include:

Sinus bradycardia. It generates an electrical charge at a slower rate than usual.

Sinus arrest. The signals from the sinus node stop and cause skipped beats.

Sinoatrial socket block. Signals to the upper chambers of the heart are slowed or blocked, causing a pause or a skipped heartbeat.

Chronotropic incompetence. Heart rate is average at rest but does not increase with physical activity.

Bradycardia - tachycardia syndrome. The heartbeat shuffles between unusually slow and fast rhythms, usually with a long pause (asystole) between beats.

WHAT MAKES SINUS MISWARD?

- Sinus node abnormalities may be due to the following:
- Age-related wear and tear of heart tissue
- Heart disease
- Inflammatory diseases are affecting the heart.
- Medicines to treat high blood pressure, including calcium channel blockers and beta-blockers.
- Medicines to treat irregular heartbeat (arrhythmias).
- Certain medications for Alzheimer's disease
- Neuromuscular disorders, such as muscular dystrophy
- Obstructive sleep apnoea
- Rare genetic mutations

RISK FACTORS ARRHYTHMIAS OF THE SINOATRIAL (SA) NODE

Sick sinus syndrome is most common in people 70 and older. Common risk factors for heart disease can increase the risk of sick sinus syndrome:

- Arterial hypertension
- High cholesterol
- Overweight
- Lack of exercise

COMPLICATIONS ARRHYTHMIAS OF THE SINOATRIAL (SA) NODE

If your heart's natural pacemaker isn't working correctly, your heart can't work as well as it should. This can lead to:

- Atrial fibrillation, the chaotic rhythm of the upper chambers of the heart.
- Heart failure
- Stroke
- Heart attack

ARRHYTHMIA OF THE ATRIOVENTRICULAR (AV) NODE

The AV node may be a small "button" of specialized cells (approximately three by 5 mm in diameter) located near the middle of the heart, on the proper angle of the atrial septum at the center of the atria and ventricles. Its function is they help mobilize the contraction of the atria and ventricles in response to the electrical signal from the heart. The AV node coordinates the moving of the electrical signal from the heart from the atria to the ventricles. The AV conduction axis is structurally complex and affects the atria and ventricles and also the AV node. Unlike the SA node, the AV node is a subendocardial structure originating in the transition zone, formed by aggregates of cells in the right posteroinferior atrium.

The superior, medial, and posterior transitional atriodal bundles converge in the compact AV node. The compact AV node (~ 1 x 3 x 5 mm) is located at the apex of Koch's triangle, which is defined by the posterior coronary sinus ostium, the anterior tricuspid annulus, and the Todaro's tendon.

The compact AV node continues as a penetrating AV bundle where it immediately passes through the central fibre body and is close to the rings of the aortic, mitral, and tricuspid valves; therefore, you are susceptible to injury as part of valve disease or its surgical treatment.

After the sinus node (located at the top of the right atrium) generates an electrical signal, it propagates through both atria, causing these chambers to beat. The AV node then "picks up" this electrical impulse and, after a short delay, allows it to pass through the ventricles.

The short delay in the electrical pulse caused by the AV node optimizes heart function. This delay allows the atria to stop beating so that the ventricles fill entirely with blood before the ventricles start to beat.

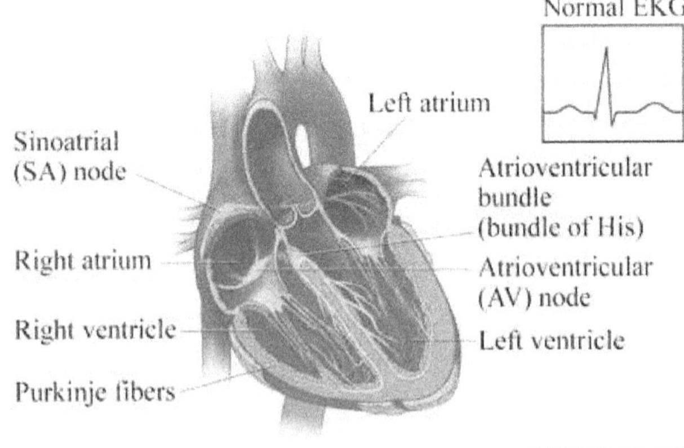

BRADYARRHYTHMIA: ATRIOVENTRICULAR NODE DISORDERS

Pulses generated in the sinoatrial (SA) node or ectopic atrial loci are directed to the ventricles through the anatomically complex electrical atrioventricular (AV) node. The electrophysiological properties of knot tissue are different from atrial and ventricular myocardium. Cells in the AV node have a relatively higher resting membrane potential than surrounding atrial and ventricular myocytes, show spontaneous depolarization during action potential phase 4, and slower phase 0 depolarization (mediated by calcium input into node tissue) than that observed in ventricular tissue (mediated by sodium influx).

Bradycardia can occur when conduction through the AV node is compromised, resulting in inefficient ventricular rates, with the possibility of associated symptoms such as fatigue, syncope, and (if secondary pacemaker activity is insufficient) even death. It is essential to recognise that with interrupted AV conduction, AS activation and atrial systole can occur at average or even accelerated rates, while ventricular activation is slow or absent.

Transient AV conduction block is standard in young people and is likely the result of increased vagal tone seen in up to 10% of young adults. Persistent AV conduction failure is definitely rare in healthy adult populations, with an estimated incidence of 200 per million inhabitants per year.

However, in the setting of myocardial ischemia, aging, and fibrosis, or infiltrating heart disease, persistent AV block is much more common.

As with symptomatic bradycardia due to AS node dysfunction, permanent pacing is the only reliable treatment for symptoms resulting from AV conduction block.

POSSIBLE UNDERLYING CAUSES OF BRADICARDIA

A full medical evaluation is needed to determine the cause of a slow heart rate. An electrocardiogram (EKG or EKG), laboratory tests, and other diagnostic studies may be performed. Possible medical causes of bradycardia include:

Bradycardia can be caused by:

- Heart tissue damage associated with aging
- Damage to heart tissue due to heart disease or heart attack
- Heart disease at birth (congenital heart defect)
- Infection of the heart tissue (myocarditis)
- A complication of heart surgery
- An underactive thyroid (hypothyroidism)
- Recurrent breathing disorder during sleep (obstructive sleep apnoea)
- Medicines, including some drugs for other cardiac arrhythmias, high blood pressure, and psychosis.

- abnormal heart rhythms
- congestive cardiomyopathy
- heart attack
- stroke
- an electrolyte imbalance
- sinus disease
- injury to the atrioventricular (AV) node

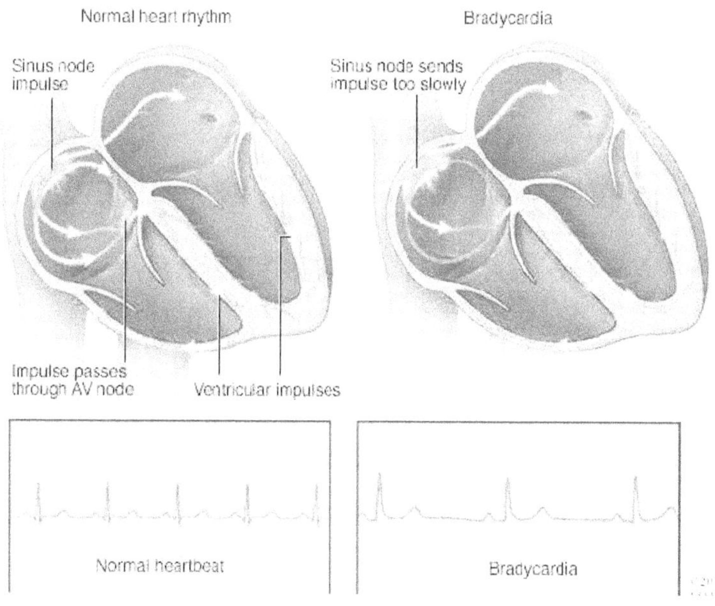

SYMPTOMS OF BRADYARRHYTHMIA

When you have bradycardia, your brain and other organs may not be getting enough oxygen, which can cause the following symptoms:

Fainting or passing out (syncope)

- Dizziness or vertigo
- tired
- Breathing problems
- Chest pain
- Confusion or memory problems
- Quickly gets tired during physical activity

TYPES OF BRADYARRHYTHMIAS

Sinus bradycardia: The heart rate is generated and executed normally, but at a rate of fewer than 60 beats per minute. It is prevalent in people without heart disease, such as athletes who exercise regularly. In general, it does not need any treatment. This can occur with sinus node disease.

Sinus Node Disease and Sinoatrial Blockages: Produced by problems in the creation of the electrical impulse in the sinus node or due to transmission from the sinus node to the atria. They usually occur in older people. If they cause symptoms, they may need to be treated with a pacemaker.

Atrioventricular blocks: They occur when the electrical stimulus is not adequately directed from the atria to the ventricles. They are classified into "first degree" (delay in impulse conduction, but none are blocked), "second degree" (some pulses are conducted, and others are blocked), and "third degree" (all are disabled). In third-degree and some second-degree cases, placement of a pacemaker is usually required. First graders generally do not need treatment. Heart blocks are classified supported the extent to which signals from the atria reach the most pumping chambers (ventricles) of the heart.

First-degree heart block: In its lightest form, all electrical signals from the atria reach the ventricles, but the signal slows down. First-degree Adams-Stokes syndrome rarely causes symptoms and typically doesn't require treatment if there are no other abnormalities in electrical signal conduction.

Second-degree heart block: Not all electrical signals reach the ventricles. Some beats "fall," resulting in a slower and sometimes irregular rhythm.

Third-degree (complete) heart block: None of the electrical impulses from the atria reaches the ventricles. When this happens, a natural pacemaker takes over, but the result is slow and sometimes unreliable electrical impulses in directing the beating of the ventricles.

ECG appearances in different types of bradycardia

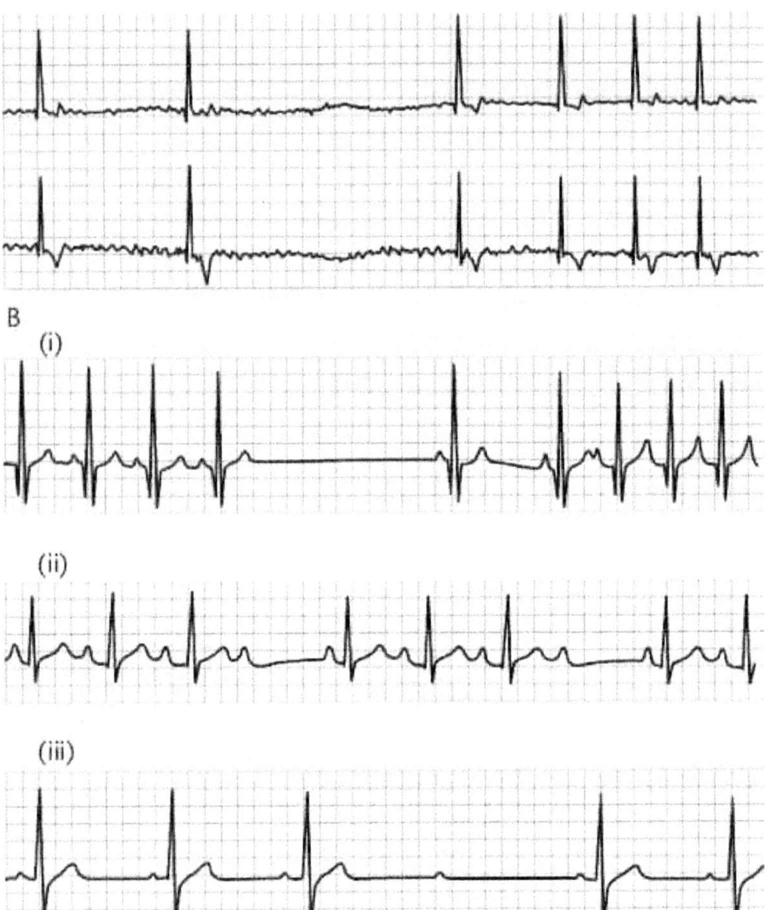

CHAPTER 10:
ATRIAL ARRHYTHMIA

Atrial arrhythmia, also known as supraventricular arrhythmia or atrial fibrillation, is an irregular and often fast heartbeat. It accelerates the risk of stroke, heart failure, and other heart complications.

In atrial fibrillation, the atria (the upper chambers of the heart) are in a state of electrical chaos, causing them to vibrate more than 600 times per minute without contracting. The lower chambers of the heart don't get regular pulses and give abnormal rhythm; hence the heartbeat turns uncontrolled and irregular. It is the deadliest atrial arrhythmia, and 75% of people who suffer from it are over the age of 60.

One of the main concerns of atrial fibrillation is the possibility of blood clots forming in the upper chambers of the heart. These blood clots that form in the heart can travel to other organs and cause a blockage in blood flow (ischemia).

Treatments for atrial fibrillation can include medications and other procedures to try to change the heart's electrical system.

TYPES OF ATRIAL ARRHYTHMIAS

- **Atrial fibrillation:** In atrial fibrillation, the atrium (the upper chambers of the heart) is in a state of electrical chaos, causing it to shake, sometimes more than 600 times per minute, without contracting. The ventricles do not receive regular pulses and act out of rhythm, and the heartbeat becomes uncontrolled and irregular. It is the most known atrial arrhythmia, and 85% of people who suffer from it are over the age of 65. Atrial fibrillation can cause a blood clot, which can enter the bloodstream and lead to stroke.
- **Premature atrial contraction:** A common and benign arrhythmia, PAC is a heartbeat that emanates from the sinus node and sends an electrical impulse through the upper chamber. It usually occurs after the sinus node starts a heartbeat and before the next regular sinus discharge. A PAC can cause a feeling of skipped heartbeats. Caffeine, tobacco or alcohol consumption, or stress, can cause or increase the frequency of NAC.

- **Supraventricular Tachycardia (SVT):** it is characterized by a fast heart rate between 100 and 240 beats per minute; SVT usually starts and ends suddenly. SVT occurs when an electrical impulse enters the atrial muscles. SVT, a condition a person can have at birth, is generally caused by a change in the heart's electrical system. SVT often starts in childhood or adolescence and can be caused by exercise, alcohol, or caffeine. SVT is rarely dangerous, but it can cause a drop in blood pressure, dizziness, or near fainting and rarely cause fainting.

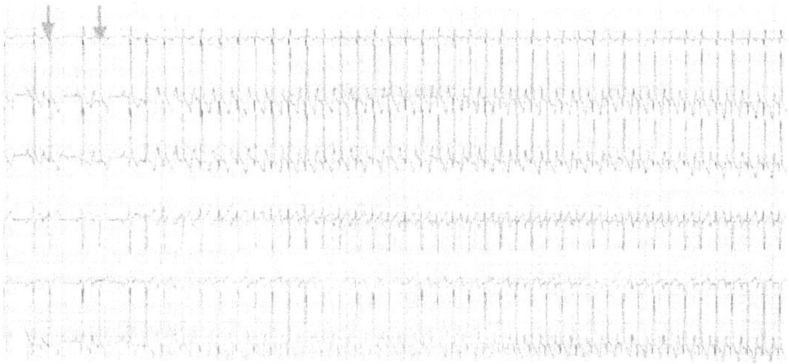

- **Atrial flutter:** Unlike atrial fibrillation because of its coordinated and regular pattern, atrial flutter is a coordinated rapid beat of the atria. Most people with atrial flutter are 60 years of age or older and have heart conditions, such as heart valve problems. As with atrial fibrillation, atrial flutter accelerates the risk of a stroke.

- **Sick Sinus Syndrome (SSS):** Common in older people, SSS is an improper activation of electrical signals caused by disease or scarring of the sinus node, sending electrical signals through the upper chamber. SSS usually slows the heart rate, but it sometimes switches between unusually slow and fast. SSS is a progressive disease, with episodes of increasing frequency and duration
- **Sinus tachycardia:** here, the sinus node sends out abnormally fast electrical signals, accelerating the heart rate from 95 beats per minute to 135 beats per minute at rest and 200 beats per minute during exercise.
- **Sinus bradycardia:** it is linked with decreased pulse generation in the sinus node; sinus bradycardia reduces heart rate to lower than 80 beats per minute.
- **Wolff-Parkinson-White (WPW) syndrome:** in WPW syndrome, an additional electrical pathway between the upper and lower chambers causes a rapid heartbeat

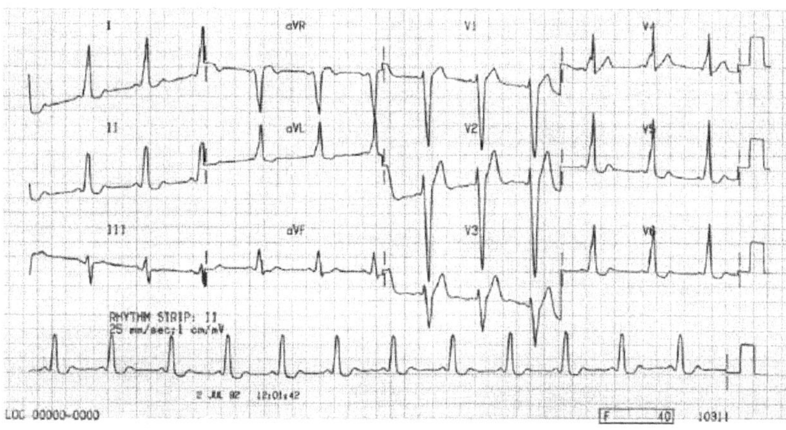

SYMPTOMS ATRIAL FIBRILLATION

Treatment of arrhythmias is recommended when it repeatedly occurs over an extended period or cause symptoms such as:

- The lightheadedness and palpitations
- Dizziness,
- Breathing problems
- Tiredness,
- Chest pain or cardiac arrest.
- Some arrhythmias can cause fainting (syncope) and sometimes a stroke, while others ("silent" arrhythmias) cause no symptoms.

Duration of arrhythmia symptoms varies depending on the type, frequency, duration, and whether or not there is structural heart disease. Arrhythmia may require medical treatment when it repeatedly occurs over an extended period of time.

Atrial fibrillation can include:

Occasionally: In this case, it is called paroxysmal atrial fibrillation (pair-ok-SIZ-mullet). Sometimes the symptoms can last up to a week, and the episodes can occur repeatedly.

Persistent: With this type, your heart rate does not return to normal by itself. If you have persistent atrial fibrillation, you will need treatment such as an electric shock or medicine to restore your heart rate.

Long persistence: This type of atrial fibrillation is continuous and lasts more than ten months.

Permanent: here, the abnormal heart rhythm cannot be reinstated. You will have permanent atrial fibrillation and often need medication to control your heart rate and prevent blood clots.

CAUSES OF ATRIAL FIBRILLATION

Atrial fibrillation is an irregular and, most time, a fast heartbeat that occurs when the two upper chambers of the heart go through chaotic electrical signals. The result is a quick and irregular heartbeat. The heart rate in atrial fibrillation ranges between 90 to 175 beats per minute. The Human Heart has four chambers: the atria and ventricles. In the upper-right section of your heart (right atrium) is a group of cells called the sinus node. It is the natural stimulator of your heart. The sinus node produces the signal that usually starts each beat.Naturally, the signal travels through the two upper chambers of the heart and then through a connecting route between the upper and lower chambers, referred to as the atrioventricular node.

The sending of the signal causes your heart to compress and sends blood to your heart and body.

The signals in the atrium of the heart are chaotic with atrial fibrillation. As a result, they vibrate. The AV node, the electrical connection between the atria and the ventricles, is bombarded with impulses that try to reach the ventricles.

The ventricles also beat fast, but not as fast as the atria because not all of the impulses pass. Damage to the structure of the heart is the most common cause of atrial fibrillation. Possible causes of atrial fibrillation include:

- Arterial hypertension
- Heart crisis
- Coronary artery disease
- Abnormal heart valves
- Heart defects you were born with (congenital)
- Overactive thyroid or another metabolic imbalance
- Lung diseases
- Previous heart surgery
- Viral infections
- Stress from surgery, pneumonia, or other illnesses
- Sleep apnoea

Here are some conditions that can lead to arrhythmia;

1. Diabetes

2. High blood pressure

3. Sleep apnoea

4. Scarring of heart tissue

5. Changes to heart structure

6. Overactive thyroid gland

7. coronary heart disease

8. Underactive thyroid gland

9. Diabetes

10. Heart attack

However, most people with atrial fibrillation don't have heart defects or damage; a condition called solitary atrial fibrillation. In isolated atrial fibrillation, the cause is often uncertain, and serious complications are rare.

ATRIAL FIBRILLATION RISK FACTORS

These include:

- **Age:** the greater your risk of developing atrial fibrillation as you age.
- **Heart disease:** Anyone with heart disease, such as heart valve problems, congenital heart defects, coronary artery disease, heart failure, or a memoir of heart attack or heart surgery, is at an increased risk of atrial fibrillation.
- **Arterial hypertension**: High blood pressure, mostly if not well controlled with medications or a good lifestyle, can accelerate your risk of atrial fibrillation.
- **Chronic conditions:** People with certain chronic conditions, chronic kidney diseases, such as thyroid problems, sleep apnoea, metabolic syndrome, diabetes, or lung disease, are at increased risk for atrial fibrillation.
- **Drinking alcohol:** Taking alcohol can trigger an episode of atrial fibrillation. Too much alcohol can increase your risk.
- **Obesity**: obese persons are at greater risk of developing atrial fibrillation.
- **Family history:** There is an increased risk of atrial fibrillation in some families.

COMPLICATIONS OF ATRIAL FIBRILLATION

Stroke: during atrial fibrillation, the chaotic rhythm can cause blood to pool in the upper chambers of the heart (atria) and form clots; it can break from your heart and travel to your brain. There it can block blood flow and lead to a stroke. The risk of stroke with atrial fibrillation depends on your age (you are at a higher risk with age) and whether you have high blood pressure, diabetes, and a history of heart failure, or stroke anterior cerebrovascular and other factors. Certain medications, such as blood thinners, can significantly reduce the risk of stroke or damage to other organs from blood clots.

Heart failure: Atrial fibrillation, mostly if left unchecked, can weaken the heart and lead to this, a condition in which your heart cannot generate enough blood to meet the need of the body.

PREVENTION OF ATRIAL FIBRILLATION

To prevent atrial fibrillation, it is essential to lead a heart-healthy lifestyle to reduce the risk of heart disease. A healthy lifestyle can include:

- Eat healthy foods for the heart
- Increase your physical activity
- Do not smoke
- keep a healthy weight
- Limit or avoid caffeine and alcohol
- Reduce stress, as intense stress and anger can cause heart rhythm problems.

- Use over-the-counter medications with caution, as some cold and cough medicines contain stimulants that can cause a rapid heartbeat.

DIAGNOSIS OF ATRIAL FIBRILLATION

Arrhythmias can be hard to diagnose because they can be unforeseeable and short. A doctor will usually take a person's medical history and perform a physical exam, where the doctor can detect arrhythmia with a stethoscope. Arrhythmias that infrequently occur last for short periods or don't cause noticeable symptoms may require more detailed tests, such as:

Electrocardiogram (ECG): This noninvasive test records the electrical activity of the heart.

Holter monitor (an ambulatory ECG): This device records cardiac activity for 24 hours or more.

Event Recorder: This portable EKG can be activated when a patient shows symptoms of a fast heartbeat. It is designed to monitor heart activity for several weeks or months.

Implantable Loop Recorder: This implantable loop recorder can be used to diagnose patients with unexplained recurrent arrhythmia episodes.

TREATMENT APPROACHES FOR ATRIAL FIBRILLATION

In some cases, arrhythmias may not need treatment. Arrhythmias causing symptoms may require one or more of the following remedies to reduce the number or duration of arrhythmic events.

- Common antiarrhythmics to suppress arrhythmias are:
- Beta-blockers,
- Calcium Channel Blockers,
- Digitalis and
- Antiarrhythmics, which affects the electrical activity of the heart.

People with atrial fibrillation have often been prescribed an anticoagulant to minimize the risk of clotting and stroke.

- **Cardioversion:** This procedure restores normal heart rhythm by sending a brief electrical shock through the chest to the heart. This restores the rhythm to normal but does not resolve underlying problems that predispose the patient to arrhythmia. Cardioversion is often used to treat:
- Atrial fibrillation
- Atrial flutter
- Ventricular arrhythmias

- **Radio-frequency catheter ablation:** For this minimally invasive treatment, a catheter with an electrode tip is placed over the affected area. The catheter supplies energy to strategically destroy tissue that disrupts the standard transmission of electrical impulses through the heart. It is most commonly used for:
    - SVT
    - Atrial flutter
    - Certain types of ventricular arrhythmias

- **Pacemakers:** This small electronic device is surgically implanted under the skin near the collarbone. The pacemaker regulates a slow or irregular heartbeat by sending rhythmic electrical charges to the right atrium and the right ventricle.
- **Maze Procedure:** For this treatment, a doctor will make several openings through the atrium. The scar tissue coordinates impulses through the heart's electrical system in a way that allows normal conduction but does not support atrial fibrillation.

CHAPTER 11: VENTRICULAR ARRHYTHMIA

An arrhythmia is a medical condition with your heart's electrical system that causes abnormal and irregular heart rhythms. Ventricular arrhythmias start in the two lower chambers of the heart, the ventricles. Usually, your heartbeat starts in the atria (upper chambers of the heart) and travels through the heart using the electrical system. Electrical signals travel through the atria, causing them to contract and pump blood into the ventricles. Then the ventricles contract to pump blood to the body.

It is a condition that occurs when the regular pattern of electrical signals is disrupted, causing the heart to beat too fast. This fast heart rate can prevent the heart from effectively pumping blood to the body. Reduced blood flow restricts oxygen supply to other organs, including the brain, which can cause fainting (syncope) and other severe symptoms.

The two most typical sorts of ventricular arrhythmias, tachycardia, and fibrillation are often life-threatening and usually require immediate medical attention.

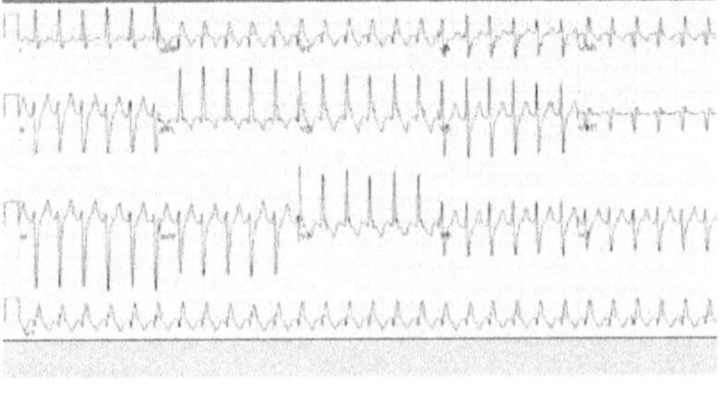

VENTRICULAR ARRHYTHMIA SYMPTOMS.

The symptoms of ventricular tachycardia (VT) and ventricular fibrillation (VFib) are similar. You may feel few or no symptoms on television, or they may come and go. With VFib, the symptoms can come on suddenly and get worse quickly.

SYMPTOMS OF BOTH TYPES OF VENTRICULAR ARRHYTHMIAS.

The symptoms of ventricular tachycardia (VT) and ventricular fibrillation (VFib) are similar. You may feel few or no symptoms on television, or they may come and go. With VFib, the symptoms can come on suddenly and get worse quickly.

Symptoms of both types of ventricular arrhythmias include:

- Chest discomfort or pain (angina pectoris)
- Fainting (syncope)
- Palpitations, feeling of palpitations
- Dizziness or vertigo
- Breathing problems

With ventricular fibrillation, a person can experience one or more of these symptoms for up to an hour before suddenly passing out or collapsing. It is ineluctable to seek immediate medical attention if any of the symptoms are detected.

Complications of ventricular arrhythmias include:

- **Organ damage**: These arrhythmias can prevent enough oxygenated blood from entering the body, which can damage the brain, kidneys, liver, lungs, and other organs.
- **Sudden cardiac arrest (SCA):** Fast and irregular heartbeat in the ventricles can cause them to vibrate unnecessarily and not pump blood. SCA can be fatal in minutes without emergency medical care.
    - Chest discomfort or pain (angina pectoris)
    - Fainting (syncope)
    - Palpitations, feeling of palpitations
    - Dizziness or vertigo
    - Breathing problems

Sustained ventricular tachycardia is recognized as follows: QRS is broad; the rate is high (> 100 bpm). It interrupts the sinus rhythm, with the first VT beat occurring before or after the P wave sine but with a shorter P-R than in the sine. The fusion of the first VT beat can occur if it occurs in a reasonable PR interval, allowing sinus conduction through with ventricular fibrillation; a person can experience one or more of these symptoms for up to an hour before suddenly passing out or collapsing. If any of these symptoms are noticed, it is essential to seek immediate medical attention.

CAUSES OF VENTRICULAR ARRHYTHMIAS.

Ventricular arrhythmias occur as a result of problems with the electrical signals that control heart rate and rhythm, such as:

- Delayed or blocked electrical signals
- Electrical signals that pass irregularly through the heart.
- Electrical signals that start outside the atria

TYPES OF VENTRICULAR ARRHYTHMIA

Arrhythmias that start in the ventricles (lower chambers of the heart) can be life-threatening and require immediate medical attention. Ventricular tachycardia (VT) can cause ventricular fibrillation (VFib).

VENTRICULAR TACHYCARDIA

This type of arrhythmia is a fast and regular heartbeat (more than 100 beats per minute) that can last a few seconds or even longer. VT prevents the ventricles from contracting entirely, which means less blood is pumped to the body. The longer the TV lasts, the higher the risk of becoming VFib. More information about ventricular tachycardia. Rapid electricity from the ventricles can cause a rapid heart rate called ventricular tachycardia or VT. With VT, abnormal electrical circuits or pathways develop in the ventricles. This can be caused by a disease that damages the heart muscle. It is most often seen after a heart attack or coronary artery disease.

The electrical signals enter the abnormal circuit and form a loop. At each loop, the signal indicates that the ventricles are contracting. It makes the heartbeat too fast to pump blood. It can cause you to pass out. In some cases, VT progresses to ventricular fibrillation. This is the deadliest type of arrhythmia because it is fatal if not treated quickly.

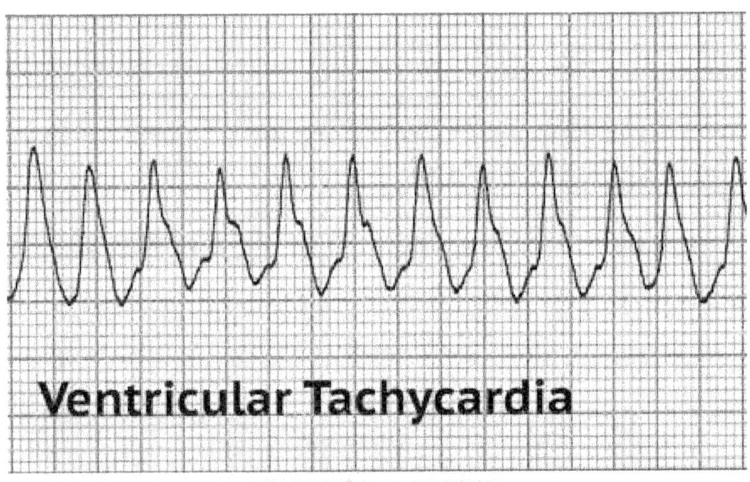

CAUSES OF VENTRICULAR TACHYCARDIA

- Severe damage to the heart
- Heart-related conditions, like cardiomyopathy, congenital heart disease, heart failure, and heart valve disease
- Heart surgery
- Lack of oxygen
- Medicines are used to treat arrhythmias.

VENTRICULAR FIBRILLATION

Sometimes electrical signals can be sent so quickly and unevenly that the heart muscle twitches and doesn't beat at all. This is called fibrillation:

VF can occur if the ventricles contain multiple abnormal circuits or if the heart muscle is seriously injured, such as from a heart attack, and becomes electrically unstable. The signals taken from the circuits cause the ventricles to beat very quickly and unevenly. This prevents the heart muscle from pumping correctly.

The heart can get so far that it cannot pump at all. This is called cardiac arrest. It will lead to death if emergency treatment is not given to return the heart rate to normal. This type of fast heart rate is very abnormal and causes the ventricles to vibrate ineffectively.

During Ventricular fibrillation, the heart cannot pump blood, resulting in a lack of oxygen to the brain and body. VFib can cause sudden cardiac arrest and death in minutes without emergency care. Read more about ventricular fibrillation.

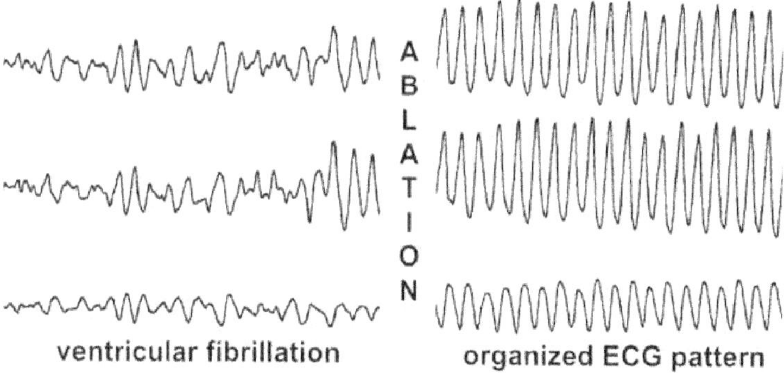

WHAT CAUSES OF VENTRICULAR FIBRILLATION

It shares some of the same causes as tachycardia, but the most known cause is a heart attack. Other causes and risk factors include:

- Some medications
- Electrocution
- Heart injury
- Narrow coronary arteries (heart)
- Torsades de pointes

Torsades de pointes is found in humans with long QT syndrome, an electrical issue that takes longer for the human heart to invigorate after each beat. It causes a rapid heartbeat, which reduces the flow of oxygenated blood. Lack of oxygen can cause sudden fainting. Brief periods of torsades de pointes can often vanish and bounce you back to responsiveness. If the conveyance takes longer, it can lead to atrial fibrillation and severe damages.

INDICATIVE TESTS FOR V A VENTRICULAR ARRHYTHMIAS

These include:

Electrocardiogram (ECG): This very test measures your heart's electrical activity for a short period of time using a monitor with electrodes placed on your body. **Electrophysiological Study:** a catheter-based test evaluates these serious ventricular arrhythmias by recording your heart's electrical signals from the human heart.

Holter and Event Monitors: these are vestments in the form of EKG monitors to ascertain the heart's electrical impulses to detect periodic arrhythmias. It continuously monitors the reading for up to 40 hours.

Implantable Loop Recorder: a small device embedded just under the skin in your chest to ascertain the electrical impulse of the heart for over a year.

TREATMENT OF VENTRICULAR ARRHYTHMIA

Things to know about Ventricular Arrhythmias:

- Premature Ventricular Contractions (PVC)
- Unsupported ventricular tachycardia
- Sustained ventricular tachycardia
- Accelerated idioventricular rhythm
- Ventricular fibrillation (VF)
- Torsades de pointes

DIAGNOSTIC CONFIRMATION

PVC is identified as a premature ventricular beat and should not be put forward by a P wave that could have been redirected (distortion of QRS). PVCs can be the same or versatile. It can be displayed alone or in batches. The origin of PVC can be ascertained by the framework of lead V1. The angle (leads 1, FAV) explains the location, such as the exit path. If the amount of PVCs is to be appraised, a Holter shot is guaranteed.

NSVT is the three consecutive PVCs but <30 seconds.

The atrioventricular (AV) node to the ventricle.

If there is AV dissociation, the diagnosis is VT. The QRS concordance, all negative (in particular) or all positive, in the precordial leads strongly suggests VT.

The appearance of R at the trough of S> 100 ms in a precordial lead also suggests VT.

Ventricular tachycardia. Take Note of the dissociation of the P waves (top band)

Other types of sustained monomorphic VT are:

Verapamil sensitive VT: This VT comes from the lower left chamber septum, and the electrocardiogram (EKG) depicts a blockage of the right beam and an upper axis. The QRS is more slender than other forms of TV.

Right ventricular (RV) VT dysplasia (ARVC): is characterized by fatty infiltration of the RV free wall. The TV shows a left bundle branch block (LBBB) pattern, and the resting sinus ECG can show a T inversion in V1-V3. There may be a notch in the QRS, the so-called epsilon waves. A variant of this condition is the RV outflow channel (RVOT) (Figure 3)/ the LV outlet channel (LVOT). This type of tachycardia has a lower axis. Most times, it can be hard to differentiate between ARVC and RVOT. QRS> 120 ms in the lead 1, earlier onset of QRS in V1, QRS notch in several leads, and favors transition from V5, V6

Recurrent bundle branch VT: is often seen in dilated non-ischemic cardiomyopathy (see below).

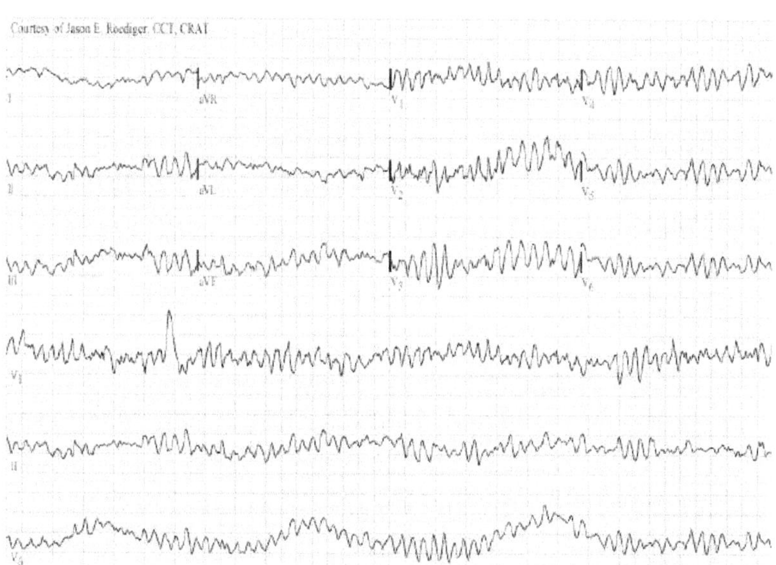

Brugada syndrome: characterized by an increase in LBBB and ST in leads V1-3.

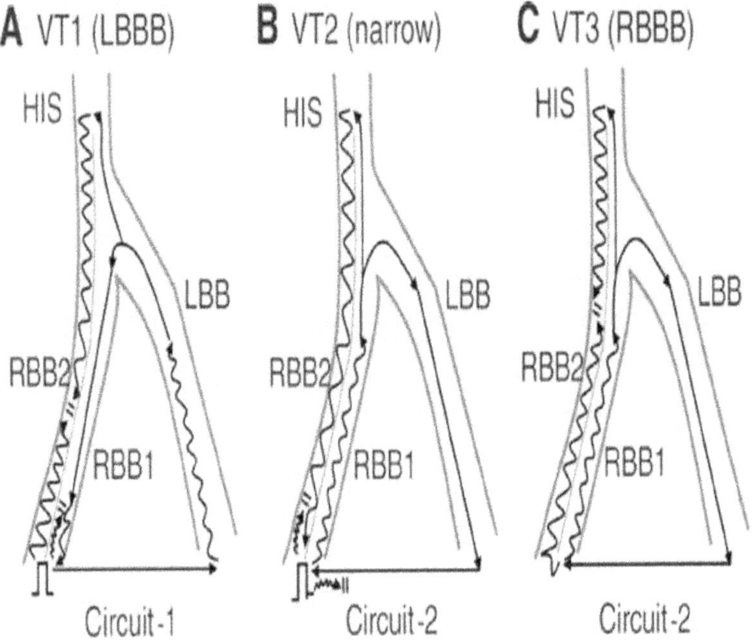

AIVR is a "slow VT" and is observed in the peri-infarct period and is defined as a VT rate <100 bpm. It can sometimes compete with the sinus beats, and fusion will occur (lead sinus beat and VT beat capturing the ventricle).

Ventricular fibrillation is at a fast and chaotic rate and should not be confused. Death is imminent. Make sure there are no artifacts in the way. In this case, careful observation will show that the QRS is running through the track and that the patient is feeling well. Early repolarization in the lower and lateral ECG leads can lead to ventricular fibrillation and sudden cardiac arrest.

Torsades de pointes is most time seen in congenital or attained Q-T syndromes but is a polymorphic VT. Other patterns of polymorphic VT with normal Q-T include CPVT (genetic defect in the ryanodine receptor of the sarcoplasmic reticulum), ischemia.

Short Q-T syndrome is a genetic condition and has been associated with sudden cardiac death.

Ventricular fibrillation is at a fast and chaotic rate and should not be confused. Death is imminent. Make sure there are no artifacts in the way. In this case, close observation will reveal the QRS running through the track, and the patient feels ok. Early repolarization in the ECG (inferior and lateral) leads can lead to ventricular fibrillation and cardiac arrest.

PATTERN RECOGNITION AND PREVALENCE

Symptoms of ventricular arrhythmias can vary based on frequency, rate, duration, and therapy. The victim may complain of palpitations, dizziness, or syncope. Sometimes flapping will be felt after PVC (e.g., Throat fullness) due to increased contraction. When it comes to therapies, beta-blockers, for example, aren't very good at suppressing PVCs, but the patient may feel less heavy. Ventricular arrhythmias may or may not be related to heart disease.

All types of ventricular arrhythmias can occur in normal and abnormal hearts. It is essential to observe the patient for the presence or absence of structural heart disease.

The following pointers can help:

- Frequent EVs in young people can be associated with mitral valve prolapse but can also be seen in normal hearts. Its density will increase with age.
- Environmental factors such as "hard" drug use and alcohol can cause these arrhythmias. Note that cardiotonic agents (oral and intravenous) can worsen ventricular arrhythmias.
- Sustained and unsupported VT could be indicative of coronary artery disease or non-ischemic cardiomyopathy. A particular type of VT in non-ischemic cardiomyopathy is bundle branch recurrence.
- Verapamil sensitive TV can be caused by exercise.
- VCs are genetic and are inherited as an autosomal dominant trait with variable penetrance.
- Torsades de pointes is linked with a long Q-T and can be acquired from drugs or inheritance. In long Q-T syndrome, women are at an increased risk of developing torsades.
- Short Q-T syndrome is genetic.
- Concurrent diagnoses that can simulate ventricular arrhythmias.

The main difference in ventricular arrhythmias is the abnormal supraventricular rhythm. Sometimes it becomes challenging to distinguish VT from an abnormal SVT.

The following tips will help you with this:

- Abnormal supraventricular rhythms are identified by P waves ahead of each QRS. Although, the Ps must be positive in leads 2, 3, and AFV, which indicates a sine origin. If P is negative, all bets are off as VT can cause 1: 1 retrograde conduction or even Wenckebach retrograde.
- The VT indices are applied, as indicated above. Nodal re-entry atrioventricular tachycardia (AVNRT), alternative atrioventricular tachycardia (AVRT), and aberrant atrial ectopic tachycardia (EAT) are preceded by negative P waves. In normal AVNRT, the P wave is usually buried in the QRS and cannot be seen.
- In AF, aberration is not uncommon, especially when the ventricular rate is high. The first broad QRS beats are usually seen after a long cycle. This is called the Ashman phenomenon. This happens because the lengthy process establishes slower conduction in the beams, with the right being lazy than the left. The next first beat is distorted (deviated) and usually in a straight beam pattern.

- In hyperkalemia, the QRS is broad, Ts peaks and P waves are absent. It's still a chest, but you can't see that Ps. Class 1 drugs such as flecainide and propafenone can increase QRS.
- Look for P waves (sinusitis, atrial flutter) that can drive the QRS. Sometimes these drugs can cause arrhythmia, and VT is possible. Wolff Parkinson White (WPW) antidromic tachycardia will present with a broad QRS. Look for P waves again.

RESULTS OF THE PHYSICAL EXAMINATION

Examine the pulse: identity as either fast or slow. Is it regular with regular irregularities? Is it irregular? In AF, there may be a gap between the apical and radial impulses.

Check the blood pressure: If it is weak, it does not help to distinguish VT from SVT. On television, pistol waves can sometimes be seen in the neck with sinus rhythm. If there are AV dissociation, fusion beats, or capture beats, S1 can vary.

WHICH DIAGNOSTIC TESTS SHOULD BE PERFORMED?

The ECG is a definitive test, and usually, arrhythmia can be easily diagnosed; that is, if a ventricular arrhythmia is detected, the presence of heart disease must be crossed out. The ECG can zoom in on the location of the PVC. Those in LV will show a model of the right bundle branch block, and those in the right ventricle will show a model of the left bundle branch block.

The axis will determine which location of the lower ventricular axis originates at the base of the heart, while an upper axis originates from the apex (see above). The stories and physics are fundamental.

A Holter image quantifies the density of the arrhythmia over a 24-hour period.

Keep in mind that high-density ventricular arrhythmias can sometimes lead to cardiomyopathy. An echocardiogram is often helpful. If there is VT, try to identify the origin: RVOT, LVOT, RV, LV, LV septum. The patient's age, history of coronary artery disease (CAD), and family history will be helpful. Coronary angiography or PE examinations are occasionally required.

HOW ARE THE RESULTS INTERPRETED?

Electrolytes are often beneficial. Check potassium and magnesium. Hypokalaemia and hypomagnesemia can be risks for torsades.

- Monitor the patient to exclude heart failure, distension of the neck vein, rheumatism, edema, etc.
- Troponins will diagnose an injury. It should be considered that in peri-infarction due to VT or VF, although the hospital death rate is higher, the long-term prognosis is ok, and there is a need to implant the implantable cardiac defibrillator (ICD).
- A regular X-ray can be useful to detect cardiomegaly, heart failure, left ventricular hypertrophy (LVH), and valve calcification.

- An echocardiogram can be very useful in determining chamber size, valve pathology, segmental wall abnormalities, HGV, septal hypertrophy, and function (ejection fraction).
- Magnetic resonance imaging (MRI) can sometimes better define structure and function, including evidence of the presence of invasive diseases such as arrhythmogenic right ventricular dysplasia (ARVD).
- Coronary angiography or perfusion imaging is suitable to include/exclude the presence of CAD.
- Electrophysiological (EP) studies are necessary for diagnostic and therapeutic reasons, especially in hypertrophic cardiomyopathy (HCM) or even Brugada syndrome. Sometimes patients with coronary artery disease, episodes of NSVT, and syncope need to be studied (see below). In the case of persistent ventricular arrhythmias induced by PE, the use of ICDs may be considered, especially in HCM.
- Mild PVCs (without heart disease) can be treated with a beta-blocker if symptomatic. Nevertheless, if the patient continues to complain even after calming down, it may be necessary to take flecainide or propafenone.

If the PVCs are from RVOT / LVOT and cardiomyopathy is present, ablation may be considered as it may be curative. Data on the definition of PVC load in this state is lacking. The idea here is that very "frequent" EVs (10% to 20% load) can compromise ventricular function over time and that drug suppression or ablation can be protective.

This is very true, especially for RVOT / LVOT PVCs. Recently, when it comes to PVC, the wider the QRS or the original shape of the epicardium, the more LV function will be restored. This is independent of the density of the PVC.

Although NSVT does not predict ejection fraction (EF) or high-density VE, it can predict future events in HCM, and ICD implantation may be warranted, especially in the presence of syncope and a positive family history of sudden death.

The presence of sustained VT depending on etiology, co-morbidity, and patient intake are essential for making the right decisions. Here are some ideas:

Hemodynamically compromised sustained monomorphic VT due to CAD is best treated with ICD, assuming revascularization is not an option. Make sure that there are no correctable conditions, such as electrolyte imbalance, ischemia, peri-infarction, or induced catheter.

The ICD won't prevent recurrent arrhythmia episodes, so amiodarone plus a beta-blocker will prevent ICD shock. Most times, it may be important to remove the TV.

RVO /LVOT: Ablation provides adequate protection without the need for antiarrhythmics

ARVC-ICD in symptomatic VT bundle branching in non-ischemic cardiomyopathy - right bundle extraction (Figure nine).

FIGURE 1

A PVC is retrograde blocked at the LBBB, transseptal to the LBBB, ascending retrograde and downstream of the LBBB, creating a continuous loop and sustained bundle branch recurrent ventricular tachycardia.

IMMEDIATE VT MANAGEMENT

Persistent VT with hemodynamic embarrassment requires immediate attention. Electrical cardioversion (EC) is required. If the patient is awake, being alert with 'good' blood pressure, intravenous medication like Lidocaine, or even synchronized EC after sedation is a good option.

Twists and turns are often self-limiting, the reason being that the tachycardia itself leads to arrest. We observe this response by accelerating the heart rate with Isuprel or pacing. A magnesium supplement is often used and can help end or prevent torsional episodes. The cause of torsades must be determined, acquired, with long-term Q-T medications (the list is very long as it includes sotalol, dofetilide, methadone, or a congenital disease), with Q-T 1-3 being the most common. The offending drug must be discontinued.

Bradycardia, if endured, is a good measure of beta-blocker activity and is considered a good prognostic sign for heart failure or in patients with a previous myocardial infarction. Other physical symptoms may not be helpful in measuring a therapeutic response.

Electrolyte disturbances are arrhythmogenic and should be monitored periodically.

Occasionally, genetic testing may be required to distinguish between types of arrhythmogenic cardiomyopathies (e.g., Brugada, long and short hereditary Q-T, ARVC, CPVT).

LONG-TERM MANAGEMENT.

Drugs associated with reducing sudden cardiac death include ASA, beta-blockers, ACE inhibitors, spironolactone, and PUFAs (polyunsaturated fatty acids). While sudden death is believed to be arrhythmic death, it may not be related.

Amiodarone and sotalol can prevent inappropriate and appropriate ICD shock.

Non-drug therapies to reduce ventricular arrhythmias include Bi-V pacing, ICD, left ventricular assistant (LVAD), coronary bypass graft (PAC), and transplantation.

COMMON MANAGEMENT PITFALLS AND SIDE EFFECTS

Medicines are challenging to take regularly. Antiarrhythmics, if successful, should not be overlooked. Note that antiarrhythmics can be proarrhythmic because they can make arrhythmia worse.

For example, flecainide and propafenone can cause sustained VT, and sotalol can cause torsades. Beta-blockers are very helpful but not without side effects such as symptomatic bradycardia, heart block, and fatigue.

All attempts must be made to ensure that the patient adheres to these medications.

Amiodarone has many side effects, including liver, thyroid, and lung toxicity, but it can suppress ICD discharges that can affect the quality of life.

Every attempt must be made at all costs to achieve the doses obtained in extensive clinical studies with positive results.

Management with co-morbidities

Diabetic statins, ACE inhibitors, and Angiotensin Receptor Blockers (ARBs) are beneficial and can affect the outcome of this condition.

ACE inhibitors, ARBs, and beta-blockers are preferred for hypertension, especially in people with kidney disease and after myocardial infarction or heart failure.

There are some restrictions on mandatory medications:

- ASA in the bleeding patient
- Spironolactone in renal failure ACEI and ARB II in acute renal failure
- Calcium channel blockers in systolic heart failure
- If necessary, stop smoking.
- Alcohol in moderation. Excess intake of alcohol can be toxic to the myocardium and cause cardiac arrhythmias (especially AF).
- Hard drugs such as cocaine can an cause acute coronary syndrome with coronary vasospasm.

- Excess caffeine can cause AF in some sensitive patients.
- Calorie restriction
- Keep calm; fear is harmful. Data on yoga and meditation may indicate beneficial effects.

QUALITY MEASURES AND PATIENT SAFETY

- Look for symptoms of dizziness, palpitations, shortness of breath, chest pain, and shock from the ICD, if applicable. ICD shocks can worsen a patient's quality of life. So look at the depression.
- Inconsistent shocks may not require further treatment, but frequent multiple shocks are indicative of antiarrhythmic therapies such as amiodarone, sotalol, and beta-blockers. Check heart rate, blood pressure, weight gain, leg swelling, and excessive sweating.
- EVs, if symptomatic, can be successfully treated with beta-blockers or flecainide, or propafenone in the absence of structural heart disease.
- NSVT may not be predictive of high PVC levels (> 10 / hr). However, in the MUSTT study, EP induces sustained VT in the presence of low EF; ICD therapy will be beneficial.

- Sustained VT often requires ICD treatment or revascularization. An ablation is an option in RVOT/LVOT; re-enter VT with a combined bundle branch.
- Amiodarone is perhaps the most potent antiarrhythmic drug to suppress all types of ventricular arrhythmia episodes.
- Intravenous verapamil may be useful in verapamil sensitive VT. Short-acting verapamil (three times a dose) is preferred for long-term treatment, as the L enantiomer (antiarrhythmic property) can escape hepatic metabolism. In sustained-release preparations, the L enantiomer is eliminated by the first-pass metabolism. Ablation is preferred.
- Torsades, if acquired, is required to omit the offending drug that could have prolonged the Q-T interval and can also provide protection.

However, sustained monomorphic VT indicates the presence of coronary artery disease. Consequently, it is reasonable to think that most ventricular arrhythmias are often associated with structural heart disease.

CHAPTER 12: JUNCTIONAL RHYTHM/ARRHYTHMIA

The SA node is the typical source of the electrical impulse of a beat. If the SA node cannot perform this function, the atrioventricular (AV) node can take over cardiac pacing. When this occurs, the ECG likely has different waveform characteristics that reveal important aspects of these junctional rhythms.

Junctional rhythm describes an abnormal cardiac rhythm resulting from pulses from a tissue locus within the area of the cardiac muscle, the "junction" between the atria and ventricles. Under normal circumstances, the heart's sinoatrial node determines how fast the organ beats; in other words, it is the "pacemaker" of the heart. The electrical activity of the sinus rhythm originates in the sinoatrial node and depolarises the atria. Current then travels from the atria through the atrioventricular node and into the bundle of His, from where it travels along the Purkinje fibers to reach and depolarise the ventricles. This sinus rhythm is important because it reliably causes the heart's atria to contract in front of the ventricles.

In the junctional rhythm, however, the sinoatrial node has no control over the heart rate; this can happen with a conduction block somewhere along the path, as explained above. When this occurs, the heart's atrioventricular node takes over like a pacemaker.

In the scenario of a junctional rhythm, the atria will contract again before the ventricles; however, this does not occur through the regular activation pathway and is somewhat due to backward conduction coming from the AV node to and through the atria. Junctional rhythms include:

- **Accelerated connection rhythm:** An accelerated junctional rhythm occurs when the AV junction triggers pulses above 60 bpm. The rhythm will be very regular. The QRS complex is narrow (0.10 s or less)
- **Junctional escape rhythm:** The joint outlet valves come out of the AV joint and are set back. The QRS complex is measured at 0.10 s or less. The rhythm is regular, with a frequency of 40 to 60 bpm.
- **Junctional tachycardia:** The abnormal rhythm arises from the bundle of His. It is seen as three or more premature junction complexes (PJC) appearing sequentially. The heart rate will be higher than 100 beats per minute.
- **Premature junction complex:** Premature junction complex (PJC) occurs when an irritable site in the AV node triggers a pulse in front of the SA node. This pulse interrupts the sinus rhythm. The QRS complex will be narrow, usually measured at 0.10 s or less.

The junctional rhythm is typical in people with sinus node dysfunction (SND), and 1 in 600 heart patients over age 65 in the United States has SND. Patients with sick sinus syndrome, young children, and athletes with an increased vagal tone may also have an intermittent attachment rhythm, especially during sleep. The percentage of unions is reported equally for men and women. Patients with a junctional rhythm can have a wide variety of symptoms, or they can be asymptomatic. The symptoms are hinged on the underlying cause of the junctional rhythm. For example, a patient with worsening heart failure may experience shortness of breath, wheezing, and lower extremity edema. Patients with rheumatic fever may have a heart murmur due to heart valve damage, fever, joint pain, and rash, with an ECG showing a junctional rhythm. Some patients may present with general symptoms such as dizziness, fatigue, syncope/presyncope, and intermittent palpitations.

Nonspecific physical examination results include pulsating veins and a steady heartbeat with a heart rate of 20 to more than 100 beats per minute.

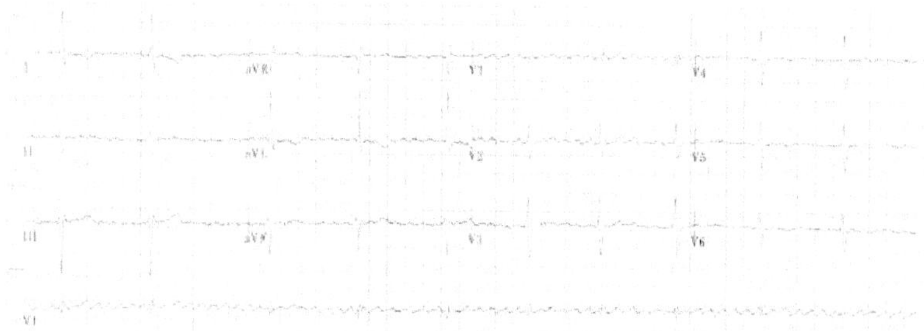

DIFFERENTIAL DIAGNOSIS

Digoxin toxicity

Nodal recurrent atrioventricular tachycardia

Recalling atrioventricular tachycardia

Sinus node dysfunction

High-quality second-degree heart block

Third-degree heart blocks

TREATMENT / MANAGEMENT OF JUNCTIONAL RHYTHM

The treatment for a binding rhythm mainly depends on the underlying cause of the rhythm. In circumstances where the junctional rhythm is the result of an underlying sinus node dysfunction leading to asystole or bradycardia, the rhythm should not be interrupted because it maintains the heart rate. Therefore, before establishing a treatment plan for patients with a junctional rhythm, an underlying etiology must be determined. Otherwise, healthy people with a binding rhythm and asymptomatic do not need medical attention, as the rhythm is usually the result of their elevated vagal tone suppressing the SA node's intrinsic automation. Due to digoxin toxicity, the patient should be treated with atropine and a specific antibody against digoxin. If a patient is refractory to these drug therapies and has junctional tachycardia, intravenous phenytoin may be administered under supervision as these patients may develop hypotension. In pediatric patients, persistent symptomatic junctional tachycardia is an indication of percutaneous radiofrequency ablation.

CHAPTER 13: COMMON CARDIOVASCULAR DISEASES

Cardiovascular disease is a health condition that is deleterious to the structures or function of the heart, such as:

ARTERIOSCLEROSIS/ATHEROSCLEROSIS

This occurs when the blood vessels that carry oxygen and nutrients from your heart to the remainder of your body (arteries) become thick and stiff, sometimes limiting the extent of blood flow to your organs and tissues. Healthy arteries are flexible and stretchy, but over time, the walls of the arteries can harden, a condition generally denoted as hardening of the arteries.

Atherosclerosis may be a specific sort of arteriosclerosis, but the terms are sometimes used interchangeably. Atherosclerosis refers to the build-up of fat, cholesterol, and other substances on the walls of the arteries (plaque), which will restrict blood flow.

Plaque can burst and cause a grume. However, atherosclerosis is usually seen as a heart problem that can affect arteries anywhere within the body. Atherosclerosis is often prevented and treated.

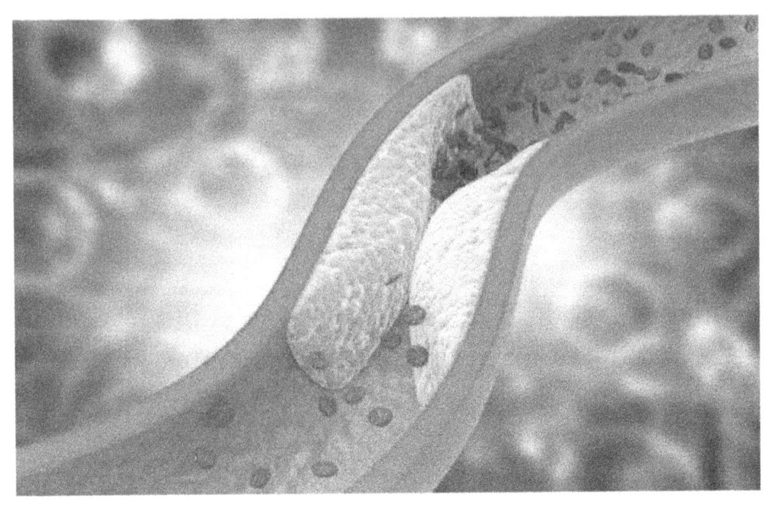

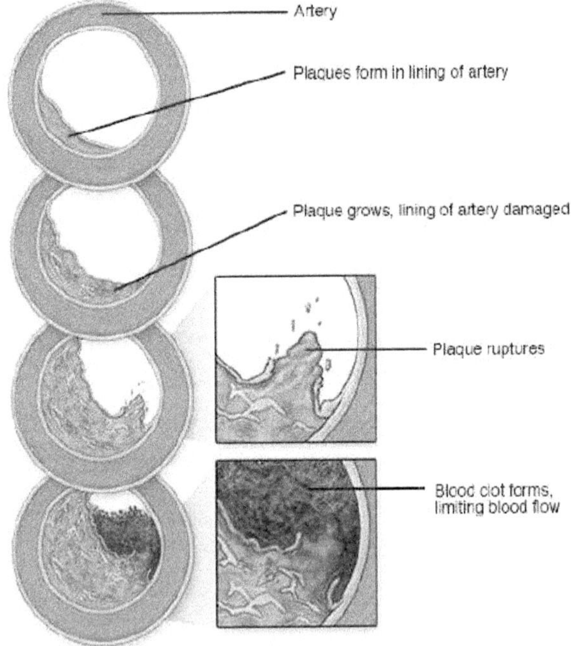
Artery
Plaques form in lining of artery
Plaque grows, lining of artery damaged
Plaque ruptures
Blood clot forms,
limiting blood flow

SYMPTOMS OF ATHEROSCLEROSIS

Atherosclerosis develops gradually. Mild atherosclerosis usually has no symptoms. You usually won't have symptoms of atherosclerosis until an artery becomes so narrowed or blocked that it cannot supply enough blood to your organs and tissues. Sometimes a blood clot completely blocks or even ruptures blood flow and can cause a heart attack or stroke. The symptoms of atherosclerosis depend on the arteries affected. For instance:

- **In the arteries of your heart**, you may experience symptoms such as chest pain or pressure (angina pectoris).
- **Around the arteries in your arms and legs**, you may have symptoms of minor vascular disease, such as pain in your legs when walking (limping).
- **Atherosclerosis in the arteries leading to the kidneys**, you will develop high blood pressure or kidney failure.

CAUSES OF ATHEROSCLEROSIS

Coronary artery disease is known to start with damage or injury to the innermost layer of a coronary artery, sometimes from childhood. It can arise from numerous factors, including:

- Refrain from smoking
- Arterial hypertension
- High cholesterol level
- insulin resistance or diabetes
- Inactive lifestyle

As soon as the inner wall of an artery is damaged, fat deposits (plaque) consisting of cholesterol and other cellular debris build-ups at the site of the injury. This process is called atherosclerosis. If the surface of the plaque tears, blood cells called platelets clump together in the place in an attempt to repair the artery. This group can block the artery and cause a heart attack.

RISK FACTORS

Risk factors for coronary heart disease include:

Age: As you age, your risk of impaired and narrowed arteries increases.

Sex: Men generally have a higher risk of coronary heart problems; nonetheless, the risk for women increases after menopause.

Family history: A family with a heart problem history has been associated with an increased risk of heart disease, especially when a close relative develops heart disease at a young age. You would be at a higher risk if your parents or siblings were diagnosed with heart disease.

- **Restrain from smoking:** People who smoke have a significantly higher risk of heart disease.
- **Arterial hypertension:** Uncontrolled high blood pressure can cause arteries to harden and thicken, narrowing the channel through which blood can flow.
- **High blood cholesterol:** High blood cholesterol can increase the risk of plaque formation and atherosclerosis. High cholesterol can be caused by low-density lipoprotein (LDL) cholesterol, also known as bad cholesterol. Low levels of high-density lipoprotein (HDL) cholesterol, called "good" cholesterol, can also contribute to the development of atherosclerosis.
- **Overweight** or Obese Being overweight tends to exacerbate other risk factors.
- **Physical inactivity:** Lack of exercise has also been linked to coronary heart disease and some of its risk factors.

- **A lot of stress:** Increased stress in your life can damage your arteries and worsen other risk factors for coronary heart disease.
- **Bad eating habits.** Refrain from eating too many foods high in saturated fat, trans fat, salt, and sugar as it can accelerate your risk of coronary heart disease.

HEART VALVE DISEASE

Heart valve disease is characterized by an injury or defect in one of the four heart valves: a mitral valve, aorta, tricuspid valve, or pulmonary.

The mitral and tricuspid valves control the movement of blood between the ventricles (the upper and lower chambers of the heart) and the atria. The pulmonary valve coordinates blood flow from the heart to the lungs, and the aortic valve ensures blood flow between the heart and the aorta, and thus the blood vessels, to the rest of the body. The mitral valve and aortic valve are usually affected by heart valve disease.

Valves that function normally ensure that the blood flows in the right direction with the right force at the right time. In heart valve disease, the valves become too narrow and hardened (stenotic) to open fully or fail to close completely (incompetence). A stenotic valve causes blood to return to the adjacent ventricle of the heart, while an incompetent valve causes blood to return to the chamber from which it previously left. To compensate for insufficient pumping action, the heart muscle gets bigger and thicker, losing its elasticity and efficiency.

In addition, the accumulation of blood in the heart chambers has a greater tendency to clot in some cases, increasing the risk of stroke or pulmonary embolism.

The severity of heart valve disease varies. In some cases, it is possible that there are no symptoms whatsoever, while in advanced cases, heart valve disease can tend to congestive heart failure and other problems. Its Treatment hinges on the extent of the disease.

Heart valve

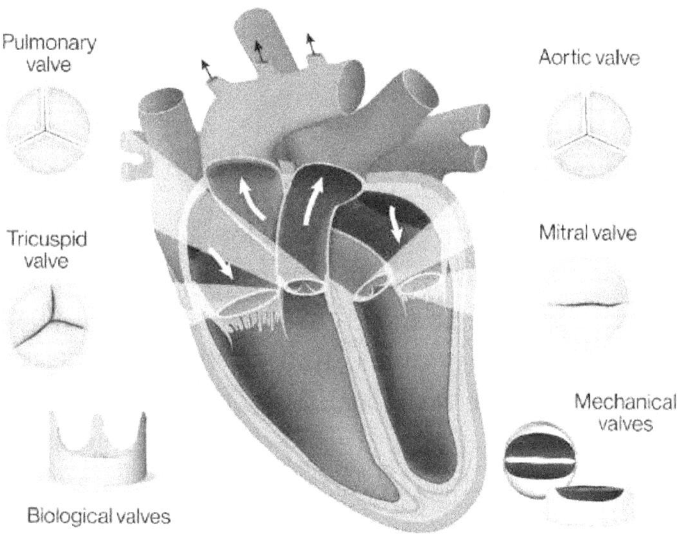

SYMPTOMS OF VALVE DISEASE

Symptoms of valve disease can come on suddenly, depending on how quickly the disease develops. As you progress slowly, your heart may adjust, and you may not easily notice these symptoms. In addition, the severity of the signs does not necessarily correlate with the severity of the valve disease. In other words, you may not have any symptoms, but you may have severe valve disease.

On the contrary, even with a small valve spot, severe symptoms can occur.

Many symptoms are synonymous with those linked with congestive heart failures, such as difficulty in breathing and swelling of the abdomen and other vital parts. Other symptoms are:

- Mild Palpitations and chest pain
- Fatigue or Tiredness
- Dizziness or fainting (with aortic stenosis).
- Fever (with bacterial endocarditis).
- Rapid weight gain

CAUSES OF HEART VALVE DISEASE

Your heart has four valves that allow blood to flow in the right way. These include the mitral valve, tricuspid valve, pulmonary valve, and aortic valve. Each valve possesses flaps (leaflets or nodules) that open and close once or twice during each heartbeat. Sometimes the valves don't open or close properly, cutting off blood flow from your heart to your body. This disease can be present at birth (congenital). It can also occur in adults due to many causes and conditions, such as infections and other heart conditions.

Heart valve problems can include:

- **Regurgitation**: In this condition, the valves do not close properly, causing blood to leak into the heart. It usually happens because of the valve flaps bulging. A condition called prolapse.
- **Stenosis:** With valve stenosis, the valve flaps become thick or stiff and can clip together. This results in a thin valve opening and reduces blood flow through the valve.

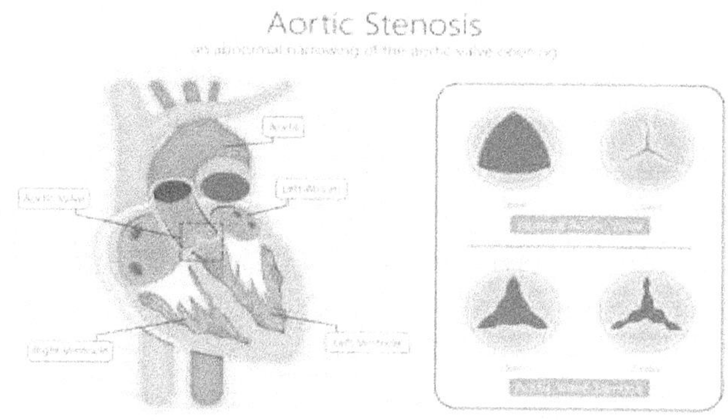

- **Atresia:** Here, the valve does not form, and a healthy layer of tissue blocks blood flow between the chambers of the heart.
- A cardiac attack can destroy the muscles that control your heart valves.

- Other conditions, such as carcinoid tumors, rheumatoid arthritis, systemic lupus erythematosus, or syphilis, can damage one or more heart valves.
- **Methysergide:** a drug used to treat migraines, and some diet drugs can promote heart valve predicaments.
- Radiation therapy (used in curing cancer) may be linked with heart valve disease.

PREVENTION OF VALVE DISEASES

Get immediate treatment for a sore throat that lasts for more than 48 hours, especially if escorted by a fever. Quick administration of antibiotics can prevent the development of rheumatic fever, which can lead to heart valve disease. A heart-healthy lifestyle is also recommended to reduce the risk of high blood pressure, atherosclerosis, and heart attack.

- Avoid smoking
- Refrain from alcohol intake.
- Eat a healthy and balanced diet reduced in salt and fat, exercise regularly, and lose weight if you are overweight.
- Follow a prescribed treatment program for other types of heart conditions.
- If you have diabetes, carefully monitor your blood sugar.

- **Do not smoke:** follow prevention tips for a heart-healthy lifestyle. Avoid excessive alcohol intake, excessive salt intake, and diet pills, all of which can raise blood pressure.
- To prevent bacterial endocarditis, a course of antibiotics is prescribed before surgery or dental work for people with heart valve disease.
- Long-term antibiotic therapy is recommended to prevent the recurrence of streptococcal infection in people who have had rheumatic fever.
- Antithrombotic (anticoagulant) medications such as aspirin or ticlopidine may be prescribed to people with heart valve disease who have had unexplained transient ischemic attacks, also called TIA.
- More potent blood thinners, such as warfarin, can be prescribed for people with atrial fibrillation (a common complication of mitral valve disease) or those who continue to have TIA despite initial treatment. Long-term administration of anticoagulants may be required after valve replacement surgery, as prosthetic valves are associated with an increased risk of blood clots.

- Balloon dilation (a surgical technique in which a small balloon is inserted into a blood vessel brought to the narrowed site by a catheter and then inflated) can be done to dilate a narrowed valve.
- Surgery of the valve may be required to repair or replace a damaged valve. Replacement valves can be artificial (prosthetic valves) or made from animal tissue (bioprosthetic valves). The type of replacement valve chosen depends on the age, the patient's condition, and the specific valve affected.

RISK FACTORS OF VALVE DISEASES

- Age factor
- Family History of certain infections that can affect the heart.
- History of some types of heart disease or heart attack.
- High blood pressure, high cholesterol, and diabetes
- Heart disease at birth (congenital heart disease)

DIAGNOSIS OF VALVE DISEASES

The doctor will listen for characteristic heart sounds during your exam, called a heart murmur, indicating heart valve disease. As part of your examination and diagnosis, you may undergo one or more of the following tests:

- **An electrocardiogram:** also called an EKG or EKG to measure the electrical activity of the heart, the regularity of the heartbeat, thickening of the heart muscle (hypertrophy), and damage to the heart muscle from the coronary artery disease.
- **Stress Test:** Also appalled as stress level test, to live vital signs, pulse, EKG changes, and rate of respiration during exercise. The heart's electrical activity is monitored by small metal sensors that are placed on your skin while you're exercising on a treadmill.
- **Chest X-ray:** echocardiogram to assess heart function. During this test, the sound waves reflected by the heart are recorded and translated into images. The pictures can reveal abnormal size, shape, and movement of the heart. Echocardiography also can be used for the calculation of ejection fraction or volume of blood pumped to the body when the heart contracts.

- **Cardiac catheterization:** Here, a catheter is inserted into the chambers of the heart to live pressure irregularities within the valves (to detect stenosis) or to watch the reflux of an injected dye on an X-ray (to detect incompetence).

CARDIOMYOPATHY

Cardiomyopathy: Maybe a progressive disease of the myocardium or cardiac muscle. In most cases, the heart muscle becomes weak and can't pump blood to the remainder of the body because it should. There are many sorts of cardiomyopathies caused by a spread of things, from arteria coronaria disease to certain medications. All of this will cause an irregular heartbeat, coronary failure, heart valve problems, or other complications.

TYPES OF MYOCARDIOPATHY

Dilated cardiomyopathy

The most known form, dilated cardiomyopathy (DCM), occurs when the heart muscle is too weak to pump blood effectively. The muscles are stretched and thin. This helps the chambers of your heart to dilate. Symptoms in babies include shortness of breath, poor appetite, and slow weight gain. Older children can also find it challenging to be physically active and become extremely tired during exercise, referred to as cardiomegaly. You'll inherit it, or it might be thanks to arteria coronaria disease.

Hypertrophic cardiomyopathy

Hypertrophic cardiomyopathy is believed to be genetic. This happens when the walls of your heart thicken and stop blood from flowing through your heart. This is often a reasonably common sort of cardiomyopathy. It also can be caused by long-term high vital signs or aging. Diabetes or thyroid disease also can cause cardiomyopathy. There are other cases whose cause is unknown. Babies with HCM often have difficulty in breathing, may sweat profusely, and have a poor appetite. Older children may have shortness of breath, fatigue, and pain. They'll also pass out or have difficulty with physical activity.

Arrhythmogenic right ventricular dysplasia (ARVD)

Arrhythmogenic right ventricular dysplasia (ARVD) may be a low sort of cardiomyopathy, but it's the leading explanation for overtime in young athletes. During this sort of genetic cardiomyopathy, fat and additional animal tissue replace the proper ventricular muscle. This causes abnormal heart rhythms. ARVC is extremely rare in children, and symptoms generally don't appear until adolescence or later.

Restrictive Cardiomyopathy

Restrictive cardiomyopathy is the least common. This happens when the ventricles become stiff and can't relax enough to fill with blood. Scarring of the heart, which is common after a heart transplant, may be the cause. It also can happen because of a heart condition.

While the symptoms of RCM are often subtle, some children can have a poor appetite, tire easily, and knowledge pain, indigestion, and a dry cough.

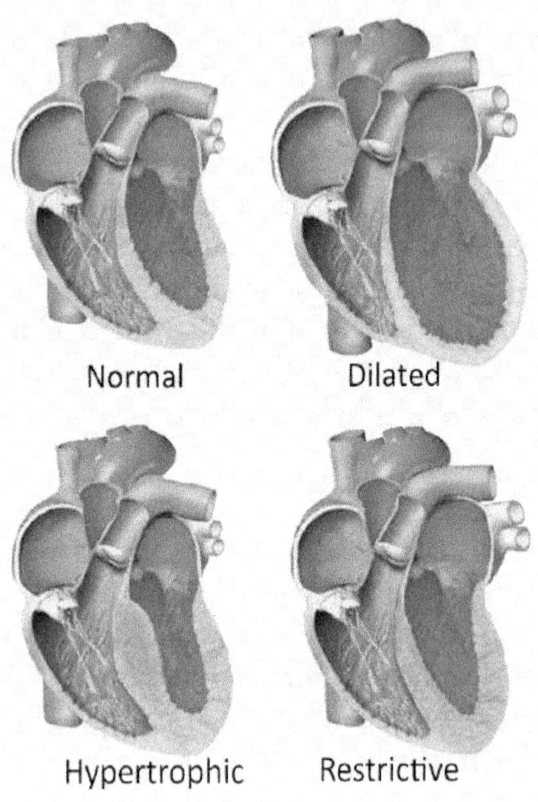
Normal
Dilated
Hypertrophic
Restrictive

Other types

Most of the subsequent sorts of cardiomyopathy fall under one among the four classifications above, but each has unique causes or complications.

- Peripartum cardiomyopathy occurs during or after pregnancy. This rare type occurs when the heart becomes weak within five months of delivery or within the last month of pregnancy. When it happens after delivery, it's sometimes mentioned as postpartum cardiomyopathy. It's a sort of dilated cardiomyopathy and a potentially fatal condition.
- Alcoholic cardiomyopathy is caused by drinking an excessive amount of alcohol over an extended period of your time, which may weaken your heart and stop blood pumping efficiently. Then your heart expands. This is often a sort of dilated cardiomyopathy.
- Ischemic cardiomyopathy occurs when your heart cannot pump blood to the remainder of your body due to arteria coronaria disease. The blood vessels of the heart muscle narrow and become blocked. This deprives the heart muscle of oxygen. Ischemic cardiomyopathy may be a common explanation for coronary failure.

  Alternatively, non-ischemic cardiomyopathy is any form not associated with arteria coronaria disease.

- Non-compacting cardiomyopathy, also called spongiform cardiomyopathy, may be a rare disease present at birth. It's the result of abnormal development of the heart muscle within the womb. Diagnosis can occur at any stage of life.

CAUSES OF CARDIOMYOPATHY

Often the explanation for cardiomyopathy is unknown. However, in some people, it's the result of another condition (acquired) or inherited from a parent (inherited).

Factors contributing to Acquired Cardiomyopathy include:

- Long-term high vital sign
- Damage to heart tissue from an attack
- Chronic fast heartbeat
- Heart valve problems
- Metabolic disorders, like obesity, thyroid disease, or diabetes.
- Nutritional deficiencies in essential vitamins or minerals, like thiamine (vitamin B-1)
- Complications of pregnancy
- Drinking an excessive amount of alcohol for years.
- Use of cocaine, amphetamines, or anabolic steroids.
- Use of specific chemotherapy and radiotherapy drugs to treat cancer.

- Certain infections, especially people who flare up the heart.
- An iron build-up within the cardiac muscle (hemochromatosis)
- A condition that causes inflammation and may cause clumps of cells within the heart and other organs to grow (sarcoidosis).
- A condition that causes the build-up of abnormal proteins (amyloidosis).
- Connective tissue disorders
- COVID-19 contamination

SYMPTOMS OF CARDIOMYOPATHY

The symptoms of all kinds of cardiomyopathy are usually similar; this will cause symptoms such as:

- general weakness and fatigue
- dizziness and vertigo
- chest pain
- Palpitations
- pass out
- arterial hypertension
- swelling of the feet, ankles, and legs

DIAGNOSIS OF CARDIOMYOPATHY

In some cases, cardiomyopathy is diagnosed when heart murmurs are detected during a routine doctor visit. However, children with cardiomyopathy may not always have a heart murmur differently to diagnose cardiomyopathy using special genetic tests, which may be done if a loved one has the disease. Unfortunately, because cardiomyopathy is difficult to detect, many children aren't diagnosed until the disease has progressed to the purpose where they show signs of coronary failure. Various tests are often used to aid in the diagnosis of cardiomyopathy and also to determine the type of disease. These include:

- Echocardiogram: This test, which helps doctors determine the type of cardiomyopathy in a child, also due to the extent of cardiac dysfunction, uses sound waves to experience the dimensions and shape of the heart and creates an image of the heart.

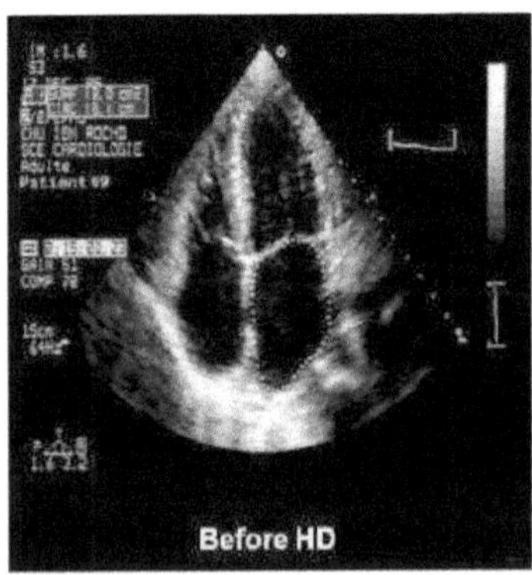

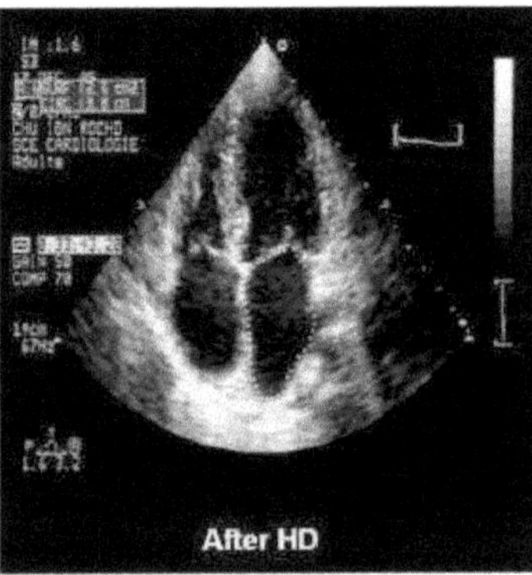

- Computer tomography (CT or CAT) or resonance imaging (MRI): These tests provide a three-dimensional image of the heart.
- Electrocardiogram (EKG or EKG): By generating a record of the heart's electrical activity, this test is frequently used to check for asymmetrical heart rhythms called arrhythmias and to prove that the heart muscle is contracted.
- Holter monitor: This is often a little portable device that's worn for 1 to 3 days and continuously records the child's pulse. It is often used to detect irregular heart rhythms often related to dilated, hypertrophic, or restrictive cardiomyopathy.
- Electrophysiology (EP) Study: Doctors insert special electrode catheters (long, flexible wires) into the veins within the groin and route them through the heart. These catheters detect electrical impulses and may even be used to stimulate different parts of the heart and map the heart's electrical system.
- Radionuclide ventriculogram: Low-dose material is injected into a vein that goes to the heart. Pictures are then crazy, a special camera, which doctors use to assess heart function.

- Cardiac catheterization: Flexible plastic tubes called catheters are inserted into a vein within the groin area then guided into the heart for a straightforward assessment of heart function. The dye is injected into the catheter to see for blocked arteries. The pressure within the chambers of your heart is often measured to ascertain how hard the blood is flowing through your heart.
- Genetic testing: Blood, tissue, and urine tests could also be done to see if your child has another genetic condition associated with cardiomyopathy. How well a toddler is diagnosed with cardiomyopathy does depend on the sort of cardiomyopathy they need and, therefore, the stage of the disease.
- Treadmill assay - Your pulse, vital signs, and breathing are going to be checked while you're walking on a treadmill. Your doctor may recommend this test to assess symptoms, determine your ability to exercise, and determine if exercise is causing abnormal heart rhythms.
- Cardiac resonance. This test utilizes magnetic fields and radio waves to make images of your heart. Cardiac MRI is often utilized in addition to echocardiography, especially if the pictures from your echocardiogram don't allow diagnosis.

- Cardiac scanner. You lie on a table during a doughnut-shaped machine. An X-ray tube within the device rotates around your body and collects images of your heart and chest to assess the dimensions and performance of the heart and its valves.
- Blood Test: A spread of blood tests could also be performed, including those used to check thyroid, kidney, and liver function and to check your iron levels.

CHEMOTHERAPY RISK FACTORS

- Several factors can increase your risk of cardiomyopathy, including:
- Family history of cardiomyopathy, coronary failure, and sudden asystole
- Long-term high vital sign
- Conditions affecting the heart, including a previous attack, arteria coronaria disease, or infection of the heart (ischemic cardiomyopathy)
- Obesity, which makes the heart work harder
- Long-term alcoholic abuse
- Use of illegal drugs, like cocaine, amphetamines, and anabolic steroids.
- Specific chemotherapy and radiotherapy drugs for cancer

- Certain diseases, like diabetes, an underactive or overactive thyroid, or a condition that causes the body to store excess iron (hemochromatosis)
- Other conditions that affect the heart, like a condition that causes abnormal protein build-up (amyloidosis), a disease that causes inflammation and may cause clumps of cells within the heart and other organs to grow (sarcoidosis), or animal tissue disorders

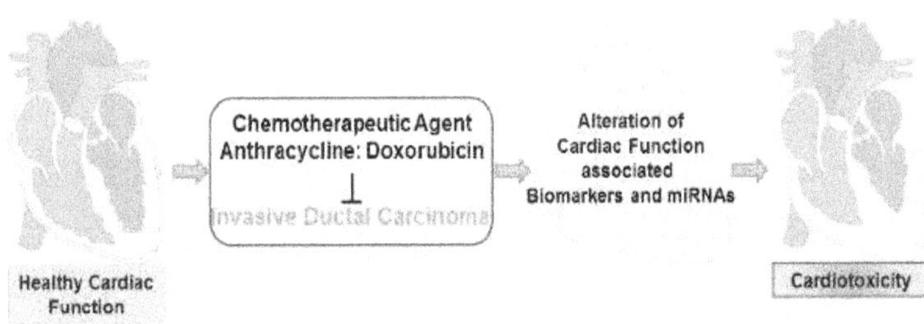

COMPLICATIONS OF CHEMOTHERAPY

Cardiomyopathy can cause other heart conditions, including:

• Heart failure. The heart cannot supply enough blood to satisfy your body's needs. If left untreated, coronary failure is often life-threatening.

• Blood clots. Because your heart cannot pump efficiently, blood clots can form in your heart. When clots enter the bloodstream, they will block blood flow to other organs.

• Valve conditions. Because cardiomyopathy makes the heart enlarge, the heart valves might not close properly. This will cause a backflow of blood.

• Cardiac arrest and overtime. Cardiomyopathy can cause abnormal heart rhythms. These abnormal heart rhythms can cause fainting or, in some cases, overtime if your heart stops beating effectively.

PREVENTION OF CHEMOTHERAPY

In many cases, cardiomyopathy cannot be prevented. Let your doctor know if you have a family memoir of the disease.

You can help reduce your risk of cardiomyopathy and other heart diseases by deciding to live a healthy lifestyle and choosing lifestyle options such as:

- Avoid the use of alcohol or cocaine.
- Maintain h*igh cholesterol*, blood pressure, and diabetes
- Healthy food

- Exercise regularly
- Get enough sleep
- Reduce your stress

CHEMOTHERAPY TREATMENT

The goal of cardiomyopathy treatment is to control your signs and symptoms, prevent your condition from getting worse, and reduce the risk of complications. Treatment depends on the type of cardiomyopathy you have. People diagnosed with cardiomyopathy often need aggressive treatment specific to the type of cardiomyopathy they have and the height of the damage to the heart.

Surgically implanted

- Numerous types of devices can be placed in the heart to improve function and relieve symptoms, including:

    - Implantable Cardioverter Defibrillator (ICD). This device monitors your heart rate and delivers electric shocks, if necessary, to control abnormal heart rhythms. An ICD does not treat cardiomyopathy but instead monitors and controls abnormal rhythms, a severe complication of the disease.

- Ventricular Aid (VAD): Helps blood flow through your heart. VAD is generally considered after the failure of less invasive approaches. Pacemaker. This tiny device placed under the skin on the chest or abdomen uses electrical impulses to control arrhythmias.

Non-surgical

- Other ways used to treat cardiomyopathy or arrhythmia includes:
    - Septal ablation. A small portion of the heart muscle is destroyed by injecting alcohol into the artery through a long, thin tube (catheter) that carries blood to that area. This allows blood to flow to the area.
    - Radiofrequency ablation. To treat abnormal heart rhythms, doctors run long, flexible tubes (catheters) through blood vessels to the heart. Electrodes at the end of the catheter transfer energy to destroy a small piece of a typical heart tissue that is causing the abnormal heart rhythm.

Surgery

The types of surgery that are used to treat cardiomyopathy include:

Septal myomectomy. In this open-heart surgery, the surgeon removes part of the thickened heart muscle septum that divides the two ventricles. Taking out part of the heart muscle enhances blood flow to the heart and reduces mitral valve regurgitation.

CHAPTER 14: AUTOMATIC NERVOUS SYSTEM

The autonomic nervous system is a collection of motor neurons that are situated in the head, neck, thorax, abdomen, and pelvis areas of the body.

The autonomic nervous system (ANS) was formerly called the vegetative nervous system. It is a division of the peripheral nervous system which helps with the smooth supply of muscle and glands. This way, it influences the function of internal organs. The autonomic nervous system (ANS) is a control system that acts chiefly unconsciously and regulates some functions in the body, which include urination, heart rate, digestion, pupillary response, and sexual arousal. This system is the primary mechanism that controls the fear or flight response in the body.

The integrated reflexes control the autonomic nervous system through the brainstem to the spinal cord and other organs.

The autonomic functions of ANS include the control of respiration, vasomotor, cardiac regulation, and some reflex actions like sneezing, coughing, vomiting, and swallowing. These are also subdivided into other areas and are associated with the peripheral nervous system and autonomic subsystems. The hypothalamus of the brain serves as the integrator for autonomic functions.

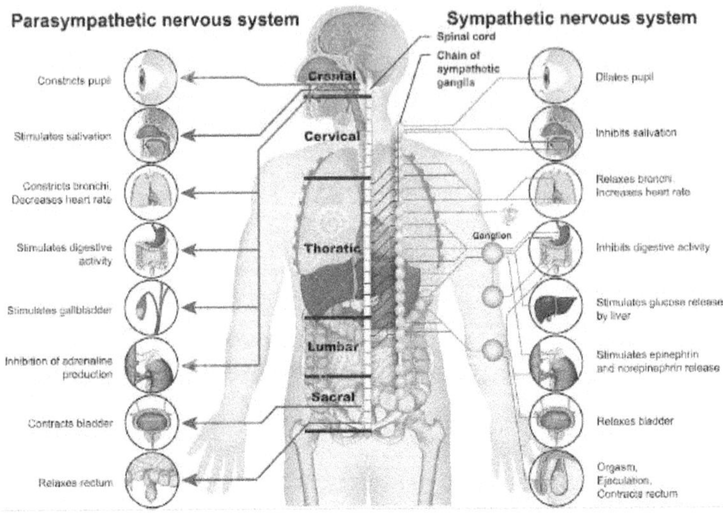

History of Autonomic Nervous System.

Traditionally, rational thought and emotional feeling have always been seen as two distinct feelings. It was believed that the brain is responsible for the rational thoughts and ideas that guide our behaviors and interactions. Emotions, on the other hand, were considered visceral and were associated with some internal organs of the body. That is why we have some figurative sayings like 'vent our spleen' and having 'gut feelings.'

Bichat divided life into two marked forms; the relational life and the organic vegetative life. The former being governed by the brain, and the latter being governed by the abdominal ganglia. The vegetative life was believed to be connected with our passions, which are governed by the abdominal ganglia, which are functioning independently.

Phillips Pinel, who was Bichat's teacher, and who was also one of the initiators of psychiatry, considered a mental disease as being caused by an abnormal function of these "little brains" (ganglia). To date, modern psychiatry still has to do with the vegetative life.

The term Autonomic Nervous System was coined by Langley, who recognized the absence of sensory nerve cell bodies in the automatic ganglia, hence defining the automotive nervous system as a motor system. He also followed that the ANS indeed does function chiefly on its own, without any interference from the central nervous system. However, Langley did not strictly follow the above simplification.

In 1903, Langley wrote in his introduction to ANS that one can consider those that give rise to reflexes in autonomic tissues and cannot independently and directly give rise to the sensation as afferent autonomic fibers.

Furthermore, the discovery of primary afferent neurons, which are also part of the autonomic nervous system, but lie outside the central nervous system, and make no direct connection with it. They also make conceiving the autonomic nervous system entirely independent and difficult.

Modern experiments have laid out that neurons in autonomic ganglia do not possess indelible discharge patterns that are sufficiently integrated to regulate physiological functions, with the possible non-inclusion of neurons in the enteric nervous system of the large and small intestines.

The typical description of hexamethonium gives a run down the state of an individual after drug-mediated separation of the autonomic nervous system from the functional control by the brain. In the same way, when brain control of spinal autonomic preganglionic neurons is removed, the cardiovascular, bowel, and bladder functions are extremely harmed. Hence the autonomic nervous system is best seen as one of the outflows in which the central nervous system controls bodily organs in a way that the autonomic nervous system may be well established.

The cardiovascular system circulates blood throughout the entire body so that oxygen and nutrients can be supplied, as well as waste being removed from the body. For each heartbeat, blood gets pumped out of the heart into the body to supply oxygen to the lungs and muscles. Heart rate is, therefore, the number of times the heartbeats per minute. It is also related to the workload that is placed on the heart when the body is resting—the heart rate when the body is resting ranges from 60 to 100 beats per minute. But if the heart rate goes higher than 100 beats, then it is suggested that the heart is working hard to get blood circulated around the body. This indicates a problem that needs to be attended to by a doctor or specialist.

Two parts of the autonomic nervous system are responsible for controlling heart rate. They are the sympathetic nervous system and the parasympathetic nervous system.

The sympathetic nervous system releases hormones that speed up the heart rate, while the parasympathetic nervous system releases acetylcholine, which slows down the heart rate. So the heart rate can be temporarily accelerated by factors like excitement, stress, or caffeine. In contrast, the heart rate can be slowed down by taking slow breaths or meditating.

When a person exercises, the heart rate definitely gets faster so long the exercise is continued. So at the beginning of the exercise, the parasympathetic stimulation is removed by the body. Consequently, the heart rate increases gradually. As the exercise continues and becomes more strenuous, the sympathetic nervous system comes in, making the heart rate faster than before.

When one participates in cardiovascular exercises continuously over time, there will be an increase in the size of the heart, an increase in the length of time it takes for the heart to be filled with blood, and an increase in contractile strength, which will lead to the heart rate becomes slower.

The slowed-down heart rate results because there is an increase in activity of the parasympathetic nervous system. Likewise, there is a decrease in the activity of the sympathetic nervous system.

Autonomic Nervous System and Cardiac Electrophysiology.

The autonomic nervous system plays a very important role in modulating cardiac electrophysiology and arrhythmogenesis. Many years of research have also helped contribute to gaining a better knowledge of the physiology and anatomy of the cardiac autonomic nervous system. These researches have also provided evidence backing up the relationship between autonomic tone and clinically significant arrhythmias. The mechanisms through which autonomic activation becomes arrhythmogenic or antiarrhythmic are complex and different for a particular arrhythmia. In atrial fibrillation, the most common triggers are simultaneously sympathetic and parasympathetic activations. On the contrary, in ventricular fibrillation in the setting of cardiac ischemia, sympathetic activation is simply proarrhythmic, while parasympathetic activation is antiarrhythmic. In syndromes of inherited arrhythmia, ventricular tachyarrhythmias and sudden cardiac death are precipitated by sympathetic stimulation.

Identifying specific autonomic triggers in different arrhythmias has brought the pattern of modulating autonomic activities for preventing and treating these cases of arrhythmias. This has been made possible by stimulation or neural ablation. In diseases like long QT syndrome, neural modulation has been established as a mode of treatment. But in other arrhythmia diseases, it is still an emerging modality that is under investigation.

William Harvey pointed in 1628 that there is a connection between the brain and the heart. He wrote that there is a cause of agitation whose effect reaches the heart when there is an affection of the mind that is attended to with pain, pleasure, fear, or hope.

For the past fifty years, a lot of anatomic and physiological studies on the cardiac autonomic nervous system have investigated this link and found that it is very complex. Not only does an autonomic activation alter the heart rate, hemodynamics, and conduction, but it also alters cellular and subcellular properties of individual myocytes.

The characterization of the extrinsic cardiac autonomic nervous system and intrinsic cardiac autonomic nervous system, ranging from recognizing the anatomic relationships at the gross level to discovering mechanoreceptors, chemoreceptors, and intracardiac ganglia, which are lining specific areas along with the cardiac chambers and great vessels.

Additionally, studies that began about 80 years ago demonstrated how critical the role of the cardiac autonomic nervous system is in arrhythmogenesis. This subject has managed to accumulate much interest due to the increasing evidence that shows that cardiac arrhythmia can be effectively controlled using neural modulation, either by stimulation or ablation.

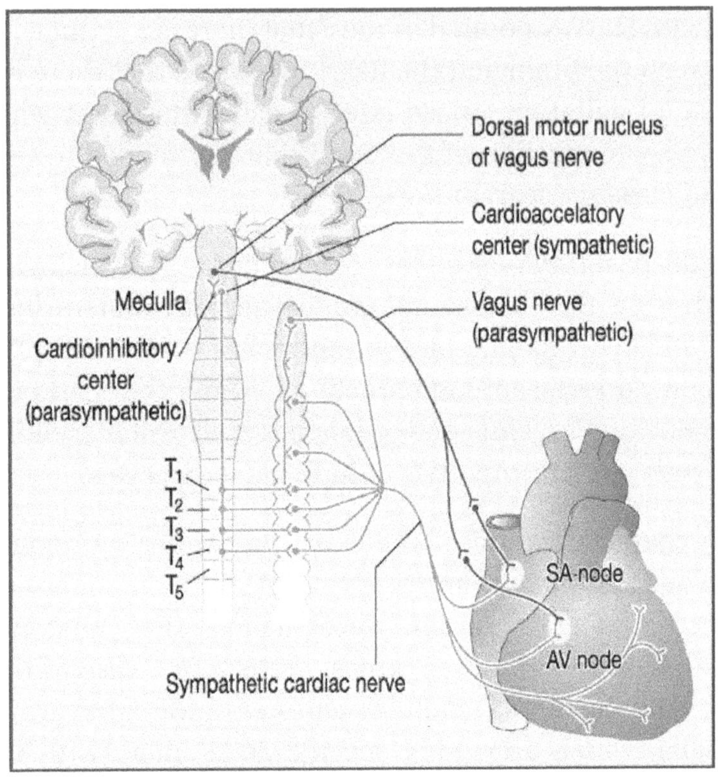

Normal Autonomic Innervation of the Heart

The cardiac autonomic nervous system can be categorised into extrinsic and intrinsic components. The extrinsic cardiac ANS is made up of fibers that act as middle connections between the heart and the nervous system, while the intrinsic cardiac autonomic nervous system has to do primarily with the autonomic nerve fibers when they enter the pericardial sac.

Extrinsic Cardiac Nervous System

This can be further subdivided into sympathetic and parasympathetic components. The sympathetic fibers are mainly gotten from major autonomic ganglia along the cervical and thoracic spinal cord. These autonomic ganglia consist of the superior cervical ganglia, which communicate with the stellate ganglia, communicates with C7–8 to T1–2, and also the thoracic ganglia. These ganglia serve as house for the cell bodies of most postganglionic sympathetic neurons whose axons form the middle, superior and inferior cardiac nerves, which terminate on the surface of the heart. The parasympathetic innervation primarily originates in the nucleus ambiguus of the medulla oblongata.

The parasympathetic preganglionic fibers are carried almost completely within the vagus nerve and are then broken down into superior, middle, and inferior branches. Most of the vagal nerve fibers combine at a distinct fat pad amidst the superior vena cava and the aorta in passage to the sinus and atrioventricular nodes.

Intrinsic Cardiac Nervous System

The heart is also reinforced by a well complex intrinsic cardiac ANS. Armour et al. showed a detailed map of the distribution of autonomic nerves in the heart of humans. Throughout the heart, there are a lot of cardiac ganglia, each of which has 200 to 1000 neurons—about 6 or 17 synapses with the sympathetic and parasympathetic fibers that go into the pericardial space.

The wide majority of these ganglia are arranged into ganglionated plexi (GP) on the surface of the ventricles and atria. In this manner, the intrinsic cardiac ANS forms a complex network that is composed of ganglionated plexi, concentrated inside epicardial fat pads, and the interconnecting axons and ganglia. These ganglionated plexi may serve as integration centers that regulate the intricate autonomic interactions between the intrinsic cardiac ANS and the extrinsic cardiac ANS. Various primary groups of ganglionated plexi have been identified in the atria and ventricles. The ganglionated plexi are concentrated on specific locations in the chamber walls in the atria. Particularly, the sinus node is basically activated by the right atrial ganglionated plexi, while the inferior vena cava innervate the atrioventricular node. The pulmonary vein is also a part that is innervated by the ANS, and it also has a high density of ganglionated plexi.

In the pulmonary vein, cholinergic and adrenergic nerves, closely located, are contained. However, the atrial ganglionated plexi may seem located in different areas on the chamber walls. The ventricular ganglionated plexi are found at the origins of various major cardiac blood vessels which surround the aortic root, the origin of the right, acute marginal coronary artery, the origin of the left obtuse marginal coronary artery, the origin of the posterior descending artery and the origin of left and right coronary arteries.

The basic characteristic of the autonomic influences on the heart is its ying-yang nature. The interaction between the sympathetic and parasympathetic nervous systems is very complex.

It was first observed in anaesthetised cats during the 1930s, Rosenblueth and Simeone, that the reduction in heart rate, which was produced by a vagal stimulus, was greater when put under tonic sympathetic stimulation.

Simeone also discovered this in anaesthetised dogs the year after. Then the term described the negative chronotropic effect of the vagal stimulation in the presence of background sympathetic stimulation as 'accentuated antagonism.'

This rare occurrence was also observed in conscious animals. Vagal antagonistic action does not only exist in chronotropic effect by opposing the sympathetic actions at the pre and postjunctional level but is also in control of cardiac electrophysiology, intracellular calcium handling, and also the control of ventricular performance.

In Chrolarose anaesthetised cats, Schwartz demonstrated that sympathetic nerve activity was reflexively inhibited by the afferent vagus nerve stimulation. Four decades later, Shen observed, by recording autonomic nerve activity in ambulatory canines, using an implanted device, that the left side cervical autonomic nervous system caused a notable reduction in the activity of the sympathetic nerve from the left stellate ganglion.

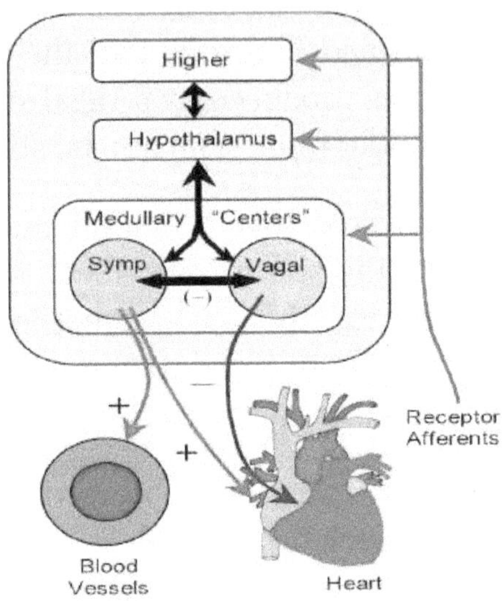

Normal Autonomic Tone in Cardiac Electrophysiology

The influences of the sympathetic nervous system on cardiac electrophysiology are complex ones and are modulated using myocardial function. With a normal heart, action potential duration is shortened by sympathetic stimulation. Also, the transmural dispersion of repolarization is reduced.

On the other hand, in pathological states like heart failure and long QT syndrome, sympathetic stimulation then becomes a potent stimulus for generating arrhythmias by enhancing the dispersion of repolarization.

Vagal stimulation does not have similar effects on the ventricular and atrial myocytes, but sympathetic stimulation does not. Vagal stimulation extends the effective refractory period and action potential duration in the ventricles.

While in the atria, the effective atrial refractory is reduced by vagal activation. Vagal activation also augments the spatial electrophysiological heterogeneity and also promotes EAD (early after depolarization) shortly before the end of phase 3 in the action potential.

The differential effect here explains why the parasympathetic stimulation is proarrhythmic in the atria and antiarrhythmic in the ventricles. In contrast, the sympathetic stimulation is proarrhythmic for the upper and lower chambers.

A technique of studying cardiac autonomic activity, which is noninvasive, is the heart rate variability analysis.

Using power spectral study of heart rate variability over a period of ECG recordings in reflecting cardiac sympathovagal balance and sympathetic tone has been used widely.

Like the heart rate variability analysis, another method that has proven noninvasive is the thorough measurement of baroreflex sensitivity. The firing of stretch-sensitive neurons which are in the afferent baroreceptor can be triggered when there is an increase in aortic volume or pressure. Then, impulses are sent to the medulla, leading to a decrease in the efferent sympathetic activity and an increase in efferent parasympathetic activity so that the pressure of homeostasis can be restored.

These analyzes give a significant prognostic value. This means that baroreflex sensitivity or depressed heart rate variability when myocardial infarction gets associated with higher cardiac mortality.

However, these noninvasive techniques have considerable limitations for at least two reasons.

1.) The analysis, instead of giving the absolute intensity of sympathetic and parasympathetic discharges, only measures the relative changes in autonomic nerve activity.

2.) In such analysis, an intact sinus node that mediates adequate cardiac responses to autonomic activity is required.

Patients with ischemic heart disease, which is a dominant risk of ventricular arrhythmias, usually suffer from associated sinus node dysfunction, hence, rendering the analysis of the baroreflex sensitivity or heart rate variability in patients with arrhythmias not unreliable.

Piccirillo showed that the correlation between actual nerve recordings and power spectral analysis is significant at baseline but not in HF. This might be as a result of the fact that there is diminished sinus node responsiveness to autonomic modulation.

The limitations listed earlier made chronic direct nerve activity recordings highly useful in demonstrating whether an autonomic activity directly triggers cardiac arrhythmias or not.

Pathophysiology of Autonomic Dysfunction in heart failure

The definite points for the sympathetic and vagal efferent discharge are changed within the central nervous system (CNS) in patients that have chronic HF. The peripheral nervous system also displays some altered responses. Basically, there is an impaired vagal nerve-controlled heart rate modulation, and augmented chemoreceptor, skeletal muscle, which is either mechanic or metabolic, and renal afferent reflexes.

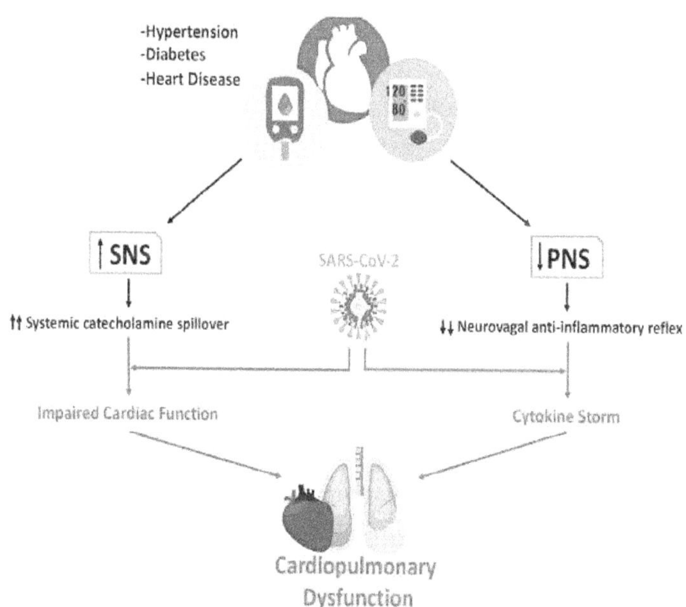

The Techniques Used in Measuring Autonomic Dysfunction in Heart Failure Patients

An objective assessment of the autonomic nervous system would be invaluable. This will not occur only in the identification of the subpopulation of patients that are diagnosed with HF and those with significant autonomic maladaptation but also when it comes to monitoring the effects of any treatments directed at the autonomic nervous system.

All the same, there are no reliable reference standards or clinically available methods that can be used to measure the functionality of the autonomic nervous system.

There are several other different techniques; each can provide a unique insight into different limbs of the sympathetic nervous system and parasympathetic nervous system, with differing strengths and limitations. These techniques can also be divided into two; non-invasive and invasive measurements.

Non-invasive techniques

An elevated resting heart rate is associated with the activation of the sympathetic nervous system and parasympathetic nervous system withdrawal. This is not only a risk marker but is a risk factor of worse prognosis in HF. When treating Systolic Heart failure, using the If inhibitor Ivabradine Trial (SHIFT), the lowest risk was marked in patients with heart rates of less than 60 beats per minute.

International guidelines favour the initiation of treatment in symptomatic HF patients, who are in sinus rhythm and have a heart rate of greater than 70 beats per minute to achieve a resting heart rate of fewer than 60 beats per minute.

The dynamic assessment of heart rate, respiratory ventilation frequency, and blood pressure provides further data on the functionality of the autonomic nervous system. How blood pressure and heart rate answer to simple maneuvres like standing (Sympathetic and parasympathetic nervous system), deep breathing (Parasympathetic nervous system), handgrip stress (Sympathetic nervous system), and Valsalva's maneuvre (baroreceptor, sympathetic and parasympathetic nervous system), are quite different in healthy individuals compared to how it is with patients diagnosed with HF. Nonetheless, none of these have proven any prognostic importance to date. However, recent data may suggest that chronotropic incompetence has some prognostic value.

The autonomic nervous system also regulates the beat-to-beat heart rate variability. Heart rate variability analysis is relatively simple to perform. It requires only consecutive RR intervals. However, there are various important impediments to its widespread adoption into clinical and academic practice. However, a reduced heart rate variability has been shown to be related to shortened survival in HF. This parameter is not a direct quantification of the activity of the sympathetic nervous system.

Also, the heart rate variability is influenced by both the sympathetic and parasympathetic nervous systems.

This includes both the pre-synaptic and post-synaptic pathways. Hence, heart rate variability will not be a specific correlate of cardiac sympathetic nervous system function.

Furthermore, as HF progresses, the analysis of heart rate variability using the conventional methods is reduced due to the presence of atrial fibrillation, frequent ectopy, and the increasing influence of respiratory rhythm-driven very low-frequency oscillations.

In patients who are still in sinus rhythm, Heart rate variability is reduced. Finally, the optimal technique for calculating heart rate variability is still not clear. Frequency domain, time domain, and non-linear analyzes of heart rate data collected in short (10 minutes) or long (24 hours) time intervals are being applied, and presently, the use of short-segment electrocardiography (ECG/EKG) for spectral heart rate variability and 25-h ECG for time-domain analyzes are well laid out. These issues raise the question of how heart rate variability may be employed effectively in patients with HF, both clinically and also for research purposes.

Heart rate alternates as a reflex response to the fluctuations of blood pressure due to the effects of baroreceptor function. Also, the lack of adequate reflex vagal activation has proven to have the best prognostic value. The sensitivity of the baroreceptor can be also be tested through interventions that can severely affect blood pressure. This includes the peripheral administration of a vasopressor or vasodilator drug or by the imposition of a mechanical stimulus. His Valsalva's maneuvre, lower body, negative pressure, and neck suction.

It is very vital to note that pressure rise quickly and primarily activates the parasympathetic limb.

On the other hand, a drop in pressure activates the sympathetic limb of the baroreceptor reflex arc. Suppose there is a continuous registration of blood pressure available together with heart rate. Also, the sensitivity of the baroreflex regulation of heart rate can be determined in a simple, automated, and non-invasive manner. This is done by calculating the slope of the regression line relating spontaneous changes that are in the RR interval to the antecedent systolic blood pressure.

A method used to assess the baroreflex, which accounts for the pressure of increased arterial wall stiffness with age, has also been well established.

The heart rate variability is greatly influenced by the Autonomic Nervous System. A lot of diseases have been associated with changes in the autonomic nervous system.

Hence, the pattern of heart rate variability is altered. Nonetheless, the variability of the heart rhythm is originated within the Sinus Atrial Node. The sinus atrial node has its own variability despite the fact that both oscillators produce heart rate variability. The influence of the sinus atrial on heart rate variability has not yet been fully studied.

https://en.m.wikipedia.org/wiki/Autonomic_nervous_system

https://www.verywellmind.com/what-is-the-autonomic-nervous-system-2794823

https://health.ucdavis.edu/sportsmedicine/resources/heart-rate.html

https://health.ucdavis.edu/sportsmedicine/resources/heart-rate.html

https://www.hindawi.com/journals/jdr/2019/5157024/

https://www.sciencedirect.com/science/article/abs/pii/0165183885900487

CONCLUSION

The 12-lead surface ECG can indicate pathological changes; structural changes within the heart are often diagnosed by other methods. The recording of an ECG was of great value for several past generations of cardiologists and continues to supply vital information. Further research is required to better explain the performance characteristics of the ECG to determine under what circumstances, if any, and these devices could precede, replace, or increase the quality of the ECG in testing strategies to detect clinically important patients within the patient population of interest. To thoroughly assess the impact of those devices on the diagnostic approach for patients with pain, test performance must be linked to clinically essential outcomes through modelling or longitudinal studies.

www.ingramcontent.com/pod-product-compliance
Ingram Content Group UK Ltd.
Pitfield, Milton Keynes, MK11 3LW, UK
UKHW021908190726
13853UKWH00002B/569